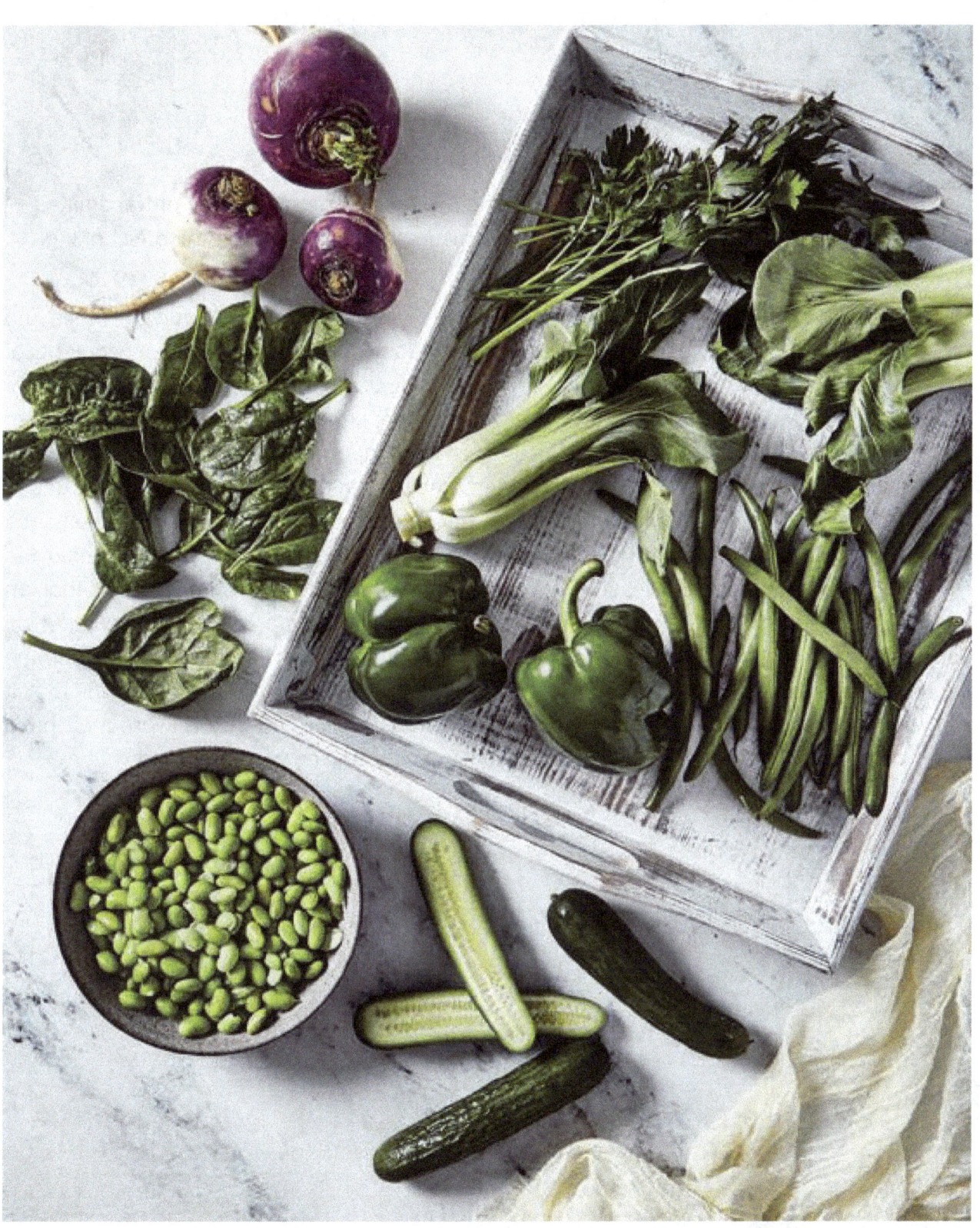

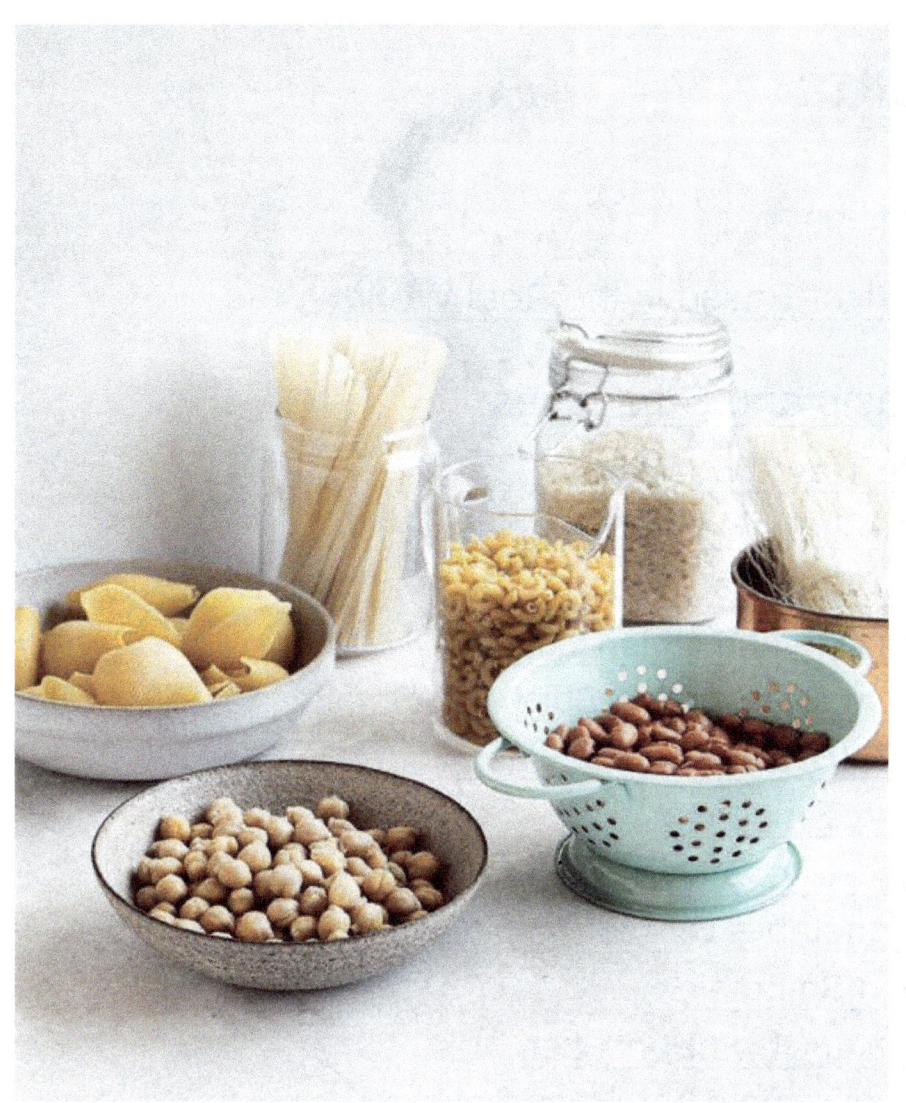

Contents

Introduction

1 Eating Plant-Based in the Real World

2 Breakfasts and Smoothies

Pancake Tray, Two Ways

Zucchini-Carrot Oatmeal Muffins

Fried "No Egg" Sandwich

Peppery Kale and Onion Scones

Mushroom and Scallion Chickpea Omelet

Smoky Barbecue Tempeh Hash

Very Berry Smoothie

Pumpkin Spice Scones

Mixed Vegetable Tofu Scramble

Go Green Smoothie

Parsley and Chive Pancakes

Sun-Dried Tomato and Basil Oatmeal

3 Salads and Bowls

Tangy Sesame Garden Salad

Spicy Italian Salad with Chickpeas

Chopped Avocado Chickpea Salad with

Olives Dill Pickle Pasta Salad

Caesar Pasta Salad

Buffalo Ranch Pasta Salad

Creamy Broccoli Slaw Salad

Spicy Chickpea Bowls

Tofu Shawarma Bowls with Pearl Couscous

Veggie Fajita Bowls

Crispy Teriyaki Tofu Vermicelli Bowls

Tempeh Bulgogi Rice Bowls

Watermelon Poke Bowls

Spicy Peanut Tofu Mango Bowls

Veggie Bibimbap

Greek Veggie Bowls with Hummus

4 Handhelds

Cheesy Summer Squash Flatbreads

Seven-Layer Burritos

Crab Cake Burgers

Veggie Supreme Garlic Bread Pizza

Cashew Curry Tofu Pita Pockets Tofu-

Lettuce-Tomato-Avocado Sandwich

Spinach and Mushroom Baguettes with Garlic-Herb Cream

Cheese Tofu Fish Tacos

Kung Pao Tempeh Lettuce Wraps

Tandoori Jackfruit and Chutney

Panini Jerk Tofu Wraps

Seitan Gyros with Tzatziki

Black Bean Meatball Subs

Pizza Pockets

5 Pasta and Noodles

Tofu Pad Thai

Creamy Garlic Penne

Tex-Mex Mac and Cheese

Pizza-Night Penne

Pad See Ew

Spinach and Ricotta Stuffed Shells

Fiery Linguini with Spinach and

Peas Curry Penne with Mango

Chutney Burst Cherry Tomato

Rigatoni Pasta Primavera

Creamy Sun-Dried Tomato and Spinach Pasta

Vegetable Lo Mein

Singapore-Style Vermicelli

Udon Noodles with Mushrooms and

Cabbage Creamy Cajun Mushroom Pasta

6 Stir-Fries and Curries

Broccoli Ramen Stir-Fry

Sweet and Spicy Tofu with Green

Beans Butter Bean Kurma

Fiery Tofu with Cashews

Vegetable Fried Rice

Red Curry Vegetables

Cauliflower, Potato, and Pea Curry

Orange Tofu

Wicked Hot Clean-Out-the-Fridge

Curry Curried Okra and Tomatoes

Kung Pao Broccoli and Cauliflower

Egg-Roll-in-a-Bowl Stir-Fry

Eat-the-Rainbow Vegetable Stir-Fry

Coconut Curry Ramen

Sweet Potato and Spinach Curry

Butter Chicken Tofu

Yellow Curried Chickpeas with Kale

Stir-Fried Teriyaki Udon Bowl

7 Soups, Stews, and Chilis

Vegetable Pho

Spicy Corn Chowder

Tortilla Soup

Broccoli Cheddar Soup

Spicy Peanut Satay Ramen

Tempeh Barbecue Chili

Lemony Split Pea Soup

Sweet Potato Coconut Curry Stew

Creamy Vegetable Soup

Chickpea and Potato Stew

Tomato Basil Gnocchi Soup

Chili Rice and Beans

Tofu Shakshuka

Creamy Lasagna Soup

Pasta e Fagioli

8 Homemade Staples

Basic Seitan

Meat-Free Pepperoni

Mango Chutney

Cheddar-Style Cheese Sauce

Vegan Mozzarella

Garlic and Herb Tofu Cream Cheese

Everyday Curry Paste

Vegan Mayonnaise

Stir-Fry Sauce

Tofu "Beef" Crumble Three Ways

Introduction

Hello! Welcome to plant-based eating for the real world. I'm assuming you're here because you're looking for an easier way to get food on the table. You've come to the right place.

There are more resources than ever for the plant-based diet, but finding the time to cook is not getting any easier. Whether it's work, kids, school, or errands, getting food on the table is hard—and it's even harder for plant-based eaters, with certain foods being quite literally off the table. Being plant-based means spending more time in the kitchen, since you can't just stop by the grocery store and hit the deli counter. It requires a bit more planning and creativity to manage a menu that isn't repetitive or boring.

As a mom with two small children, I find that life is constantly busy. Getting a nutritious, balanced, plant-based meal on the table day after day is challenging. I often find I'm short on time for meal prep—and dinnertime has a habit of constantly sneaking up on me. When my family switched to a plant-based diet almost a decade ago, there wasn't much available in terms of convenience foods. Now, mainstream grocery stores and even restaurants are stocked with plant-based options and products, but they come with big trade-offs from both a health and financial perspective.

My goal with this book is to show you that it is possible to cook a wide variety of healthy, delicious plant-based meals using real ingredients, in less time than it takes for restaurant delivery. Whether you're new to plant-based eating, you're a seasoned vegan, or you want to add a little more veg into your omnivore diet, you'll find recipes in this book that are full of bright, bold flavors, familiar ingredients, and easy-to-follow directions.

At the beginning of this book, I'll walk you through some plant-based cooking basics like how to stock your refrigerator and pantry with some key ingredients. I'll show you shopping shortcuts and other time-saving hacks (meal planning is your friend here) and explore some of the must-have kitchen tools to make your life easier. We'll also cover some of the benefits of healthy plant-based eating for you and your family.

The recipes in this book are broken down into categories based on the type of meal you're looking to make, from breakfast to dinner. I've chosen favorites of mine that use minimal ingredients but yield maximum flavor, that can often be cooked in one pot (to keep cleanup easy), and that take you on a culinary journey around the world. Dishes like Creamy Sun-Dried Tomato and Spinach Pasta, Butter Bean Kurma, Tex-Mex Mac and Cheese, Tofu Shakshuka, and Vegetable Pho will soon become your favorites, too.

So, toss those takeout menus in the trash—let's get cooking!

1

Eating Plant-Based in the Real World

Plant-based eating is becoming more mainstream every day. Both sit-down and quick-serve restaurants are catering to plant-based eaters with varied menu options; food manufacturers are developing and launching new plant-based meats and dairy alternatives, and the whole plant-based movement is gaining worldwide momentum. This makes shopping for and cooking vegan dishes much easier than it's ever been.

That all being said, plant-based eating does require a little more preparation and planning than omnivore cooking does. There aren't really as many "cheats" in the plant-based cooking realm as there are in omnivore diets. Replicating meat-based proteins in plant-based dishes is easy to do, but it requires some additional prep and cooking time. In this book I'll share tips and tricks for making plant-based versions of your favorite dishes in record time.

The Plant-Based Diet

Healthy plant-based cooking can be a challenge at the best of times. Add in the challenge of a busy schedule, and, well . . . it can be downright exhausting.

The truth is that plant-based eating does require more time and planning. There is no "grocery store rotisserie chicken" substitute in the plant-based world. Most of what we cook has to come from scratch, and that takes time. But simple tricks and certain tools can help you get meals on the table in just minutes. In this chapter, I'll walk you through all of them.

But first, what exactly are we talking about with "plant-based"?

I'm defining plant-based eating as recipes that are:

- made entirely from plants (no animal products or by-products)
- as close to "whole food" as possible (with a few exceptions)
- low in salt/sugar/saturated fat

The recipes in this book use ingredients derived from plants to make tasty, nutritious meals for the entire family. I focus predominantly on fresh, whole foods, which is why I've included a chapter on Homemade Staples. There you'll find homemade versions of common "meat" substitutes, such as meat-free pepperoni and tofu "beef" crumble, so you don't have to rely on store-bought versions, which tend to be less healthy. But if time is a bigger priority, do what works best for you. We'll get into that more later in this chapter as well.

My hope is that this book will arm you with enough tips and tools to shop for and easily prepare fresh, vibrant plant-based meals that will keep you satisfied.

Plant-Powered Benefits

There are many wonderful benefits to adopting a plant-based diet, some of which you'll notice in just a few days of eating an animal-free diet. Aside from the obvious benefits to animals and to the environment, many people choose to follow a nutrient-rich, non–processed plant-based diet because of the benefits to their overall health and well-being.

» **Better mood.** Plants make people happy! Did you know that plant-based diets are rich in brain-friendly vitamins like folate and B6, which boost your mood? Plant-fueled meals also give you more energy (and don't weigh you down), so you feel like getting up and being more active.

» **Lower blood pressure and cholesterol.** Plant-based meals made from scratch (not using processed, prepackaged foods) are much lower in salt and fat, both of which contribute to high blood pressure and high cholesterol. High levels of cholesterol can cause a buildup in your arteries, leading to heart disease and stroke.

» **No more sugar crashes.** Want to keep from hitting that 3:00 pm brick wall? A diet rich in fruits, vegetables, and nuts helps keep your blood sugar levels more even, which keeps you from craving that chocolate bar and avoids the sugar high—and crash afterward.

» **Plants help you lose weight.** Avoiding sugar- and salt-laden processed foods is good for everyone, regardless of their diet, but a plant-based diet rich in vegetables, fruits, beans, and legumes gives your body the nutrients it needs without storing extra fat. You'll have more energy, which can help in your quest to burn calories and drop pounds.

Plant-Based Meals in 30 Minutes

In this book, you'll find recipes that are healthy and balanced, taste great, and can be made in 30 minutes or less. I've applied several different strategies to ensure these recipes not only take less than half an hour to prep and cook, but also use a wide variety of ingredients and flavors.

For those who are new to plant-based eating, I've developed recipes that are familiar, like macaroni and cheese, meatball subs, and teriyaki stir-fry, but with a plant-based twist, so that you can get comfortable with using plant-based ingredients and still feel like you're eating all your favorite dishes. I'll show you how to make some basic components that can be used throughout the book to add variety to your meals.

Seasoned plant-based eaters will enjoy this book for its unique look at ingredients and ways to shake up your recipe rotation by creating meals like savory [Sun-Dried Tomato and Basil Oatmeal](#), [Crab Cake Burgers](#) made from hearts of palm, [Watermelon Poke Bowls](#), [Tandoori Jackfruit and Chutney Panini](#), and more.

Cooking in under 30 minutes means getting creative about what you cook and how you prepare it—like letting your appliances run double-duty. I'm all about maximizing time and space, which means if we can get two pots on a stove cooking at once or something in the microwave, let's do it. The hardest part about cooking a variety of vegetables for one dish is that they all have different cooking times, so preparing vegetables in a way that gets them all cooked at the same time is important. The best way to do this is to keep all your vegetables the same size or to lightly steam larger, denser vegetables (like sweet potatoes, squash, or broccoli) in the microwave before adding to a pan or pot, so that they all cook in the same amount of time.

Seven Key Plant-Based Ingredients

There's nothing more frustrating than finding a recipe you'd like to make and then realizing you have to hunt all over town trying to find the ingredients for it. All the recipes in this book use ingredients that can be found in most mainstream grocery stores. But I also recommend keeping these staple ingredients on hand for quick and easy plant-

based cooking.

- » **Nutritional yeast.** Nutritional yeast is a deactivated yeast that is used to add both cheesy and nutty flavors to plant-based dishes. It's very high in protein and vitamin B and is a staple for making vegan cheeses or adding a cheesy flavor to sauces and soups.

- » **Coconut milk.** I highly recommend having a couple of cans of coconut milk in your pantry at all times. Canned coconut milk is made from two ingredients, coconut and water, and is the easiest way to make creamy curries, soups, and stews without adding any dairy. I recommend using full-fat coconut milk for cooking. Light coconut milk has most of the coconut stripped out, leaving it very thin and watery. It's like the plant-based equivalent of "skim milk."

- » **Vegetable broth.** Making your own homemade broth is always best, but it's not always convenient. I like to keep a couple of containers of low-sodium vegetable broth on hand. It's a great way to add flavor to rice or quinoa (cooking grains in vegetable broth instead of water is one of my go-to flavor tricks), and it's a great alternative to oil for sautéing aromatics.

- » **Beans and legumes.** One of the healthiest ways to add fiber and protein to your diet is to use beans or legumes. Canned chickpeas, beans, and lentils are a quick win in this department. Since they are precooked, they can be used straight from the can and just warmed up in dishes. Always choose no-salt-added versions if available.

- » **Nut butters, seed butters, and tahini.** They aren't just for PB&J sandwiches! All-natural nut or seed butters are great additions to sauces, dips, and dressings and add great flavor. Tahini (and other seed butters) are a great allergen-free way to add nutty flavors to foods.

- » **Grains and pasta.** White and brown rice, quinoa, couscous, whole-wheat noodles, and pastas are staples of many diets, and particularly helpful for plant-based diets. Keeping these staples on hand means you're always only a few minutes away from making healthy veggie-packed bowls or meals.

» **Canned tomatoes and vegetables.** I'm a huge proponent of "fresh is best," and will always opt for fresh vegetables in season. But canned vegetables, picked at the peak of their harvest, are great ways to quickly add extra vitamins and fiber to your dishes. Canned tomatoes are the backbone of so many dishes, and even a can of corn or peas and carrots can elevate a dish quickly and help you achieve those "5 servings a day."

Shopping Shortcuts

Along with the key ingredients above, I'll use this section to explore other plant-based ingredients worth adding to your regular shopping list and talk about some shortcuts I use to make shopping and cooking easier.

Tofu and Tempeh

Because animal sources of protein are not an option, having these plant-based protein substitutes on hand makes it easy to ensure you're preparing well-balanced meals. I recommend using extra-firm tofu, which has less water than softer tofu and requires less time for draining and pressing before using.

Tempeh is a pressed soy product, much like tofu but yet completely different. While tofu is made from soy curds, which are slightly more processed, tempeh uses the whole soybean, which is pressed into a block shape and naturally fermented.

The bacteria used to ferment tempeh is incredibly gut-friendly, and tempeh is generally much less processed than tofu, making it a healthier option.

Spice and Herb Blends

This is a fantastic way to add a lot of flavor to a dish while minimizing the number of ingredients used. Spice and herb blends are also great space-savers for kitchens with small storage spaces. I always recommend having a few different blends on hand. My favorites include:

- **Italian seasoning:** This blend includes herbs like basil, oregano, thyme, rosemary, and sage.
- **Curry powder:** A mild yellow curry powder adds incredible flavors to dishes. Curry powders are made up of multiple spices and vary in intensity from mild to hot. A basic mild curry powder will contain a mix of ground turmeric, chiles, cumin, coriander, ginger, and pepper. Some curry mixes include cinnamon, cardamom, and mustard seed as well.
- **Tex-Mex or chili powder:** This spicy mix contains dried chiles along with garlic, onion, and cumin and is a must-have for flavoring Tex-Mex-inspired dishes.

Frozen Assets

Nothing says "quick prep" quite like a bag of frozen vegetables.

All the peeling, chopping, and dicing is done for you, meaning you just need to open the bag and stir. I rely heavily on frozen vegetable staples in this book where possible to help keep your prep to a minimum. Mixed vegetables, like carrots, peas, corn, and green beans are always handy for boosting the veggie content in soups and stews. Frozen broccoli and cauliflower make it incredibly easy to add these nutrient-dense vegetables to stir-fries or other dishes, and if chopping onions makes you cry, you can even get frozen diced onions, which can be used in practically every recipe in this book.

Pre-Chopped Everything

I love kitchen prep. To me, it's a way to get lost in a task and decompress. There is something almost rhythmic about dicing vegetables. But it takes a long time. Taking advantage of fresh, pre-chopped vegetables or pre-spiralized noodles from your grocer's produce department is a great way to ensure you've maximized your veggie intake without logging hours in the kitchen. This goes for jarred aromatics as well, like garlic and ginger. If you have the time to mince garlic or grate ginger, by all means, do so. But if you're in a hurry, it's much easier to add a teaspoon of jarred minced garlic or grated ginger to add aromatic flavor to your dishes. I promise no one will know!

Oil-Free Hacks

Oils add caramelization and flavor and are helpful in crisping up tofu, but consuming too much oil is unhealthy. If you're making the effort to eat a plant-based diet, keeping it low-oil or oil-free will help you reap the most benefits.

When I recommend an oil in this book, I opt for grapeseed or extra-virgin olive oil. Both are lighter oils that have high smoke points (they can cook at high temperatures, so your food cooks quicker and doesn't have to "sit" in the oil).

Many readers may wish to eliminate oil from their diet. For any recipes in this book that require sautéing or caramelizing aromatics, or for quick pan-cooking vegetables, try using low-sodium vegetable broth or water in place of oil. You will need double the amount of broth/water than oil, and you'll need to keep a close eye on your pan (and lower your heat a little bit).

Time-Saving Techniques

This book is all about maximizing your meals while minimizing your prep and cooking time. To help achieve that, I've chosen similar staple ingredients for many dishes that you can buy in bulk and prepare in advance to help decrease the amount of time you need to spend in the kitchen at mealtime.

I like to prepare many staple ingredients on the weekend— usually after a grocery run—and store them in the refrigerator so they are ready to go when I need them throughout the week. Try these simple prep tips to make weeknight cooking easier.

Quick Veggie Prep

I go through a lot of bell peppers in a week, so I like to batch-prep them at the beginning of a week. I seed and cut my peppers into wide strips and store them in an airtight container in the refrigerator. This way, I can easily chop or dice a couple of strips when needed.

Having carrots peeled (and even chopped) in the refrigerator is super helpful in shortening mealtime prep, not to mention handy when you want to grab a quick snack to go with some hummus or dip. Whole peeled carrots can last in the refrigerator in an airtight container or a resealable bag for up to 5 days. To keep them extra fresh, wrap them in a damp paper towel before placing in a bag or container. Every time you grab a carrot, change the paper towel.

Everything from scallions to fresh herbs can be fabulous aromatics for dishes, but having to wash and prep them adds time to your already rushed schedule. When you bring these bright greens home from the supermarket, wash them and stick them in a glass of water on your windowsill. Don't have space in your kitchen? Wrap them in a slightly damp paper towel and store in the refrigerator in a resealable bag. The paper towel will keep them just moist enough to ensure they don't dry out.

Cooking Grains

Many grains easily cook in time to be included in a 30-minute recipe, but sometimes space can be a limiting factor or, if you're newer to cooking, it can be intimidating to have to manage multiple pots and pans—not to mention cleanup takes longer.

Batch cooking grains for the week is a great way to ensure you always have rice or quinoa ready to go at mealtime. Brown rice in particular is a great dish to prep in advance, because it often requires a longer cook time. I recommend choosing one or two grains per week, and cooking a few batches on a Sunday afternoon. Try cooking them with low-sodium vegetable broth instead of water to add flavor. Store cooked grains in an airtight container in the refrigerator and gently reheat in the microwave (adding a splash or two of low-sodium broth or water to help rehydrate them) while you cook the rest of your meal.

Health vs. Convenience

Life is about balance, and preparing fast plant-based meals often means trying to balance health with convenience. While it is, of course, much easier to grab a package of processed, plant-based meat crumbles at the grocery store and make a quick spaghetti dinner, it's not the healthiest option. But making that same dish with a tofu "beef" crumble involves many ingredients and more than 30 minutes to prepare. So, I've tried to find ways to strike that balance in this book by providing a healthy, low-prep homemade version, or the option to use store-bought convenience items, or to batch-cook/prep ingredients in advance that can be used in a dish later that week.

When writing this book, I created recipes that use fresh whole ingredients, but that also rely on a little bit of convenience through the use of oil, soy sauce, dressing, or other staples to add bright, bold flavors to these dishes. In the long run, maintaining a healthy attitude about food involves balance; flavor is just as important as health since if the dish you're making is bland, you're going to be tempted to reach for that stack of takeout menus again. In many recipes throughout the book, I've highlighted both homemade and store-bought options for ingredients like mayonnaise, curry paste, dairy-free cheeses, and more so that you can choose which options work best for you. I've also included a recipe for Tofu "Beef" Crumble Three Ways, which can be adapted to make a Tex-Mex-style crumble for the ultimate taco night, a Korean barbecue-style tofu that works incredibly well in a "beef" and rice bowl or as a filling for lettuce wraps, and of course, a Bolognese-style crumble when you're absolutely craving a huge bowl of spaghetti.

Convenient Plant-Based Tools

A well-stocked kitchen isn't limited to just food. Having the right equipment on hand will make your prep go much more smoothly and will help get you excited to get in the kitchen and start cooking. I'm not a huge gadget girl, and I don't like my kitchen being overrun with tons of equipment, so I try to focus on keeping pieces that will get the most use and make the most sense for me. Below I've recommended some key kitchen gadgets that are worth having around. I've left out the obvious, like pots, pans, and baking sheets, because those are items commonly found in most kitchens, and you can adapt what you have on hand to work for this book.

Essential Equipment

Sharp knives: When it comes to plant-based ingredient prep, which involves a lot of chopping, slicing, and dicing, a set of really good knives is worth splurging on. One solid chef's knife and a smaller paring knife are invaluable tools that will make your food prep so much easier.

Vegetable peeler: Whether you choose the standard shape (that resembles a paring knife) or a Y-shaped peeler, a handheld vegetable peeler is an absolute necessity for ensuring you can make quick work of peeling vegetable skins without peeling off half the vegetable too.

Metal colander or strainer: This is used for draining pasta (either grain-based or spiralized veggie noodles), for easy rinsing and cleaning of vegetables, and for making a quick makeshift steamer basket, which you'll need to make my [Basic Seitan](). Choose a metal version over plastic, as you can't set a plastic one over boiling water.

Blenders: Yes, I said blenders, plural. If budget and space allow, having both a high-speed upright blender and a handheld stick blender is ideal. The upright blender is perfect for making the smoothies in the breakfast chapter, and for homemade staples like [Vegan Mayonnaise]() and [Cheddar-Style Cheese Sauce](). A handheld (or immersion) blender makes pureeing soups much easier. Handheld blenders are relatively inexpensive and allow you to achieve a smooth, creamy consistency in a flash—and with less cleanup than an upright blender, since you can use a handheld blender directly in the cooking pot (just take the pot off the heat first).

Large cutting board: I have several sizes of cutting boards in my kitchen. My favorite is an 11-by-18-inch bamboo board that is solid enough to handle tons of chopping and dicing and sits flush on my counter without slipping.

Gadgets for People Who Hate Prep

Food processor: While technically you could just use a blender for any recipe in this book that requires a food processor, it is handy to have one around if your budget and space allow for it. Food processors come with multiple blades that can perform many different functions, like chopping, blending, shredding, and slicing. A standard 14-cup food processor can get you through just about any amount of kitchen prep.

Vegetable chopper and/or a mandoline: If a food processor is out of your budget, opt for smaller, manual tools like a hinged vegetable chopper and a mandoline. Both of these can easily cut vegetables, and a vegetable chopper can even dice onions, causing you fewer tears.

Microplane grater or a box grater: Both are perfect for zesting lemons and limes. A box grater has the added bonus of having four different size grating panels, meaning you can shred carrots or vegan cheese on it as well.

Plant-Based on the Fly

Thirty-minute meals are fantastic, but sometimes life gets so busy that you need something faster that still gives you the energy and nutrients you crave. These are a few of my tips for ensuring you're always ready to make a quick plant-based meal.

Keep bowl staples on hand. Having a container of precooked rice, quinoa, or even lentils in the refrigerator—or a bag of prewashed lettuce—means you always have the base for a quick and easy plant-based bowl. Toss in some prepped veggies (remember that "Time-Saving" tip above about pre-chopping all your vegetables and storing them in the refrigerator), or open a can of beans or chickpeas; add a drizzle of tahini or store-bought dressing and a handful of nuts and you've got a powerhouse meal that took just a few minutes to make.

Hummus to the rescue. Hummus is incredibly easy to make and lasts for days in the refrigerator. Toss a drained can of chickpeas, 2 tablespoons of lemon juice, ½ teaspoon each of salt and ground cumin, and 2 tablespoons of tahini in a food processor with ⅓ cup of the liquid from the chickpea can and process for 2 minutes. Now you've got a great oil-free spread for a sandwich or a wrap, or a snack with some precut vegetables.

Store-bought fallbacks. Pizza is great in a pinch, but delivery isn't always quick or healthy. Keep a whole-wheat or cauliflower pizza crust in your freezer (and a jar of tomato sauce in the pantry) and you're just a few minutes away from your own personal pie.

Upcycle your leftovers. Taco night is a standing tradition in our house, and we always have leftovers. Grab some large tortillas and fill them with leftover taco fillings (beans, rice, Tex-Mex tofu crumble, and veggies make fantastic burritos). Wrap them up, cover in plastic wrap and aluminum foil, and place in a resealable freezer bag. When hunger strikes, simply unwrap, microwave for 2 minutes, and you've got lunch. Try this with a tofu scramble, too, for breakfast burritos on the go.

About the Recipes

In this book you'll find 100 recipes for dishes that are well balanced, nutritious, and full of flavor, and that can be made in less than 30 minutes, including prep time. To help make this book easier to use, I've labeled each recipe with important details that will help you choose the recipes best suited to your dietary needs or time constraints.

For example, I've highlighted easy recipes as follows:

- **One pot:** Recipes that use only one main vessel for cooking, like one pot, one pan, or one tray. These recipes are fabulous for keeping cleanup to a minimum.
- **Superfast:** Recipes that can be made in 15 minutes or less, meaning that even on your busiest days, you can still get them on the table in time for dinner.
- **No cook:** Recipes that do not require the use of an oven, stove, or microwave.
- **Easy prep:** Recipes involving less than 5 minutes of prep time.

I've also added dietary labels to call out dietary restrictions such as:

- Gluten-free
- Nut-free

- Soy-free

- Oil-free

If buying premade items, such as vegan cheese, always check the ingredients list for any allergens.

2

Breakfasts and Smoothies

Pancake Tray, Two Ways

Zucchini-Carrot Oatmeal Muffins

Fried "No Egg" Sandwich

Peppery Kale and Onion Scones

Mushroom and Scallion Chickpea Omelet

Smoky Barbecue Tempeh Hash

Very Berry Smoothie

Pumpkin Spice Scones

Mixed Vegetable Tofu Scramble

Go Green Smoothie

Parsley and Chive Pancakes

Sun-Dried Tomato and Basil Oatmeal

Pancake Tray, Two Ways

PREP TIME: 10 minutes

COOK TIME: 15 minutes

SOY-FREE

SERVES 8

My kids call this "cake for breakfast." I call it working smarter, not harder. We have a tradition of pancakes on Saturday mornings in my house, but sometimes I don't feel like standing over the stove flipping individual cakes. This method bakes an entire pancake sheet all at once that you can cut and serve. It's also a great make-ahead dish that you can prep the night before to bake in the morning.

For the base

Cooking spray

2 tablespoons ground flaxseed

¼ cup hot water

2 cups all-purpose flour

3 tablespoons sugar (for sweet versions; reduce to 1 tablespoon for savory variations)

1 teaspoon baking powder

½ teaspoon salt

1 cup unsweetened almond milk

2 tablespoons vegetable oil

For the chocolate peanut butter version

3 tablespoons creamy peanut butter

3 tablespoons chocolate syrup

For the cheesy herb version

3 tablespoons nutritional yeast

2 tablespoons chopped fresh dill

2 tablespoons chopped fresh flat-leaf parsley

1 teaspoon onion powder

½ cup shredded Cheddar-style vegan cheese, for topping (optional)

To make the base

1. Preheat the oven to 350°F. Spray a 9-by-13-inch baking dish with cooking spray to coat the bottom and sides.

2. To make the base, in a small bowl, combine the ground flaxseed and water with a fork to form the flax eggs. Set aside.

3. In a large bowl, whisk together the flour, sugar, baking powder, and salt.

4. Add the flax eggs, almond milk, and vegetable oil and stir until a batter forms.

To make the chocolate peanut butter version

1. Pour the batter into the prepared baking pan.

2. Put the peanut butter in a small bowl and microwave it in 10-second intervals until runny but not bubbling over. For most standard microwaves this should take about 20 seconds.

3. Randomly place teaspoon-sized drops of peanut butter over the top of the pancake base. Repeat with the chocolate syrup. Using the tip of a knife or a cake tester, lightly swirl the drops together to form a marbled effect.

4. Bake for 15 minutes, or until the top is set. Remove from the oven, let sit for 5 minutes, then cut into squares and serve.

To make the cheesy herb version

1. Add the nutritional yeast, dill, parsley, and onion powder to the batter.

2. Pour the batter into the prepared baking pan. Sprinkle with the cheese (if using).

3. Bake for 15 minutes, or until the top is set. Remove from the oven, let

sit for 5 minutes, then cut into squares and serve.

VARY IT: Try swapping the chocolate syrup for some melted strawberry or raspberry jam for a PB&J pancake. Or use bananas and chocolate chips, fresh blueberries and peaches, or apples and cinnamon.

Chocolate Peanut Butter

PER SERVING: Calories: 230; Fat: 8g; Protein: 5g; Carbohydrates: 35g; Fiber: 2g

Cheesy Herb

PER SERVING: Calories: 188; Fat: 5g; Protein: 5g; Carbohydrates: 31g; Fiber: 2g

Zucchini-Carrot Oatmeal Muffins

PREP TIME: 10 minutes

COOK TIME: 20 minutes

OIL-FREE, SOY-FREE

MAKES 12 MUFFINS

As a mom, I'm always looking for ways to sneak veggies into my kids' meals. Muffins are an excellent way to do that. My kids think they're just getting a delicious treat, but I know they're also getting a serving of veggies. This recipe uses flaxseed and applesauce as binders, which adds extra fiber and vitamin C and keeps these muffins oil-free.

1½ cups all-purpose flour

½ cup rolled oats

½ cup sugar

1 tablespoon baking powder

¼ teaspoon salt

¼ cup hot water

2 tablespoons ground flaxseed

1 cup unsweetened almond milk

1 cup grated zucchini

1 cup shredded carrots

¼ cup unsweetened applesauce

1. Preheat the oven to 350°F. Line a standard muffin tin with paper liners or grease well.

2. In a large bowl, combine the flour, oats, sugar, baking powder, and salt.

3. In a medium bowl, whisk together the hot water and flaxseed, then add the almond milk, zucchini, carrots, and applesauce. Whisk to combine.

4. Pour the wet mixture into the dry mixture and stir until just combined and no flour streaks are left behind.

5. Using a 2-inch ice cream scoop (or a ¼-cup measuring cup), evenly divide the batter into the prepared muffin tin. Bake for 20 minutes, or until a toothpick inserted in the center of a muffin comes out clean.

SMART SHOPPING: Shorten your prep time by using pre-shredded carrots and spiralized zucchini. Most grocery stores sell zucchini spirals in the produce section. Simply dice up enough to fill one cup and save the rest for pasta night.

PER SERVING (1 MUFFIN): Calories: 119; Fat: 1g; Protein: 3g; Carbohydrates: 25g; Fiber: 2g

Fried "No Egg" Sandwich

PREP TIME: 10 minutes

COOK TIME: 10 minutes

NUT-FREE

SERVES 6

This recipe recreates the taste (but not the look) of a fried egg with only 10 ingredients, and in less than 10 minutes.

1 cup cold water

¼ cup nutritional yeast 1

tablespoon cornstarch

½ teaspoon ground turmeric

½ teaspoon garlic powder ½

teaspoon onion powder

¼ teaspoon paprika

1 (14-ounce) block firm or extra-firm tofu, drained and pressed

1 tablespoon vegan butter

6 English muffins, toasted and buttered

1. In a small bowl, combine the water, nutritional yeast, cornstarch, turmeric, garlic powder, onion powder, and paprika. Whisk until smooth. This is the vegan "yolk." Set aside.

2. Halve the tofu so that you have two square blocks. Turn each block on its side and slice into 3 or 4 even slices, depending on how thick you want the tofu egg. If you like, you can use a cookie cutter or the top of a cup to cut the slices into circles.

3. In a large sauté pan or skillet, melt the butter on medium-high heat. Add the tofu slices, being careful not to crowd them (you might need to do this in two batches depending on the size of your skillet). Cook the tofu for 2 to 3 minutes on each side, until lightly golden.

4. Add the vegan yolk to the pan and toss the tofu slices to evenly coat them. Cook for 3 to 4 minutes, until the yolk thickens. Transfer the

tofu slices to the prepared English muffins, drizzle with the remaining sauce from the pan, and serve.

MAKE IT AHEAD: For easy weekday mornings, make a batch of the fried tofu eggs to keep in the refrigerator in an airtight container. Reheat them in the microwave for 1 minute while you toast an English muffin, and you've got a hearty breakfast to go.

PER SERVING: Calories: 236; Fat: 6g; Protein: 14g; Carbohydrates: 30g; Fiber: 4g

Peppery Kale and Onion Scones

PREP TIME: 10 minutes

COOK TIME: 20 minutes

NUT-FREE

MAKES 12 SCONES

I've taken my basic buttermilk scone recipe and turned it into a savory breakfast scone with just the right amount of peppery heat. I've used granulated onion to simplify this recipe, but if you have the extra time, try dicing up half of a small onion and sautéing it with the kale before adding it to the scone dough.

1 cup unsweetened soy milk

1 tablespoon freshly squeezed lemon juice

3 cups all-purpose flour

1 tablespoon sugar

2½ teaspoons baking powder

2 teaspoons freshly ground black pepper

2 teaspoons granulated onion or 1 teaspoon onion powder

½ teaspoon baking soda

½ teaspoon salt

¾ cup cold vegan butter, cut into 1-inch

cubes 3 cups stemmed and shredded kale

1. Preheat the oven to 425°F. Line a rimmed baking sheet with parchment paper and set aside.

2. In a glass, combine the soy milk and lemon juice and let stand for 5 minutes to create a buttermilk substitute.

3. In a large bowl, combine the flour, sugar, baking powder, pepper, granulated onion, baking soda, and salt.

4. Using a pastry cutter if you have one (or two knives working in a crisscross cutting motion if you don't), cut the butter into the dry

mixture and mix until you have small bits of butter throughout, creating a crumbly texture.

5. Add the shredded kale and the buttermilk and stir until a dough is formed.

6. Scoop 12 even amounts of dough, about the size of tennis balls, onto the prepared baking sheet, about 1 inch apart, and bake for 17 to 19 minutes, or until golden. Serve immediately.

VARY IT: Add 1 cup vegan Cheddar-style shreds to this recipe to make cheesy onion and kale scones.

PER SERVING (1 SCONE): Calories: 229; Fat: 12g; Protein: 4g; Carbohydrates: 26g; Fiber: 1g

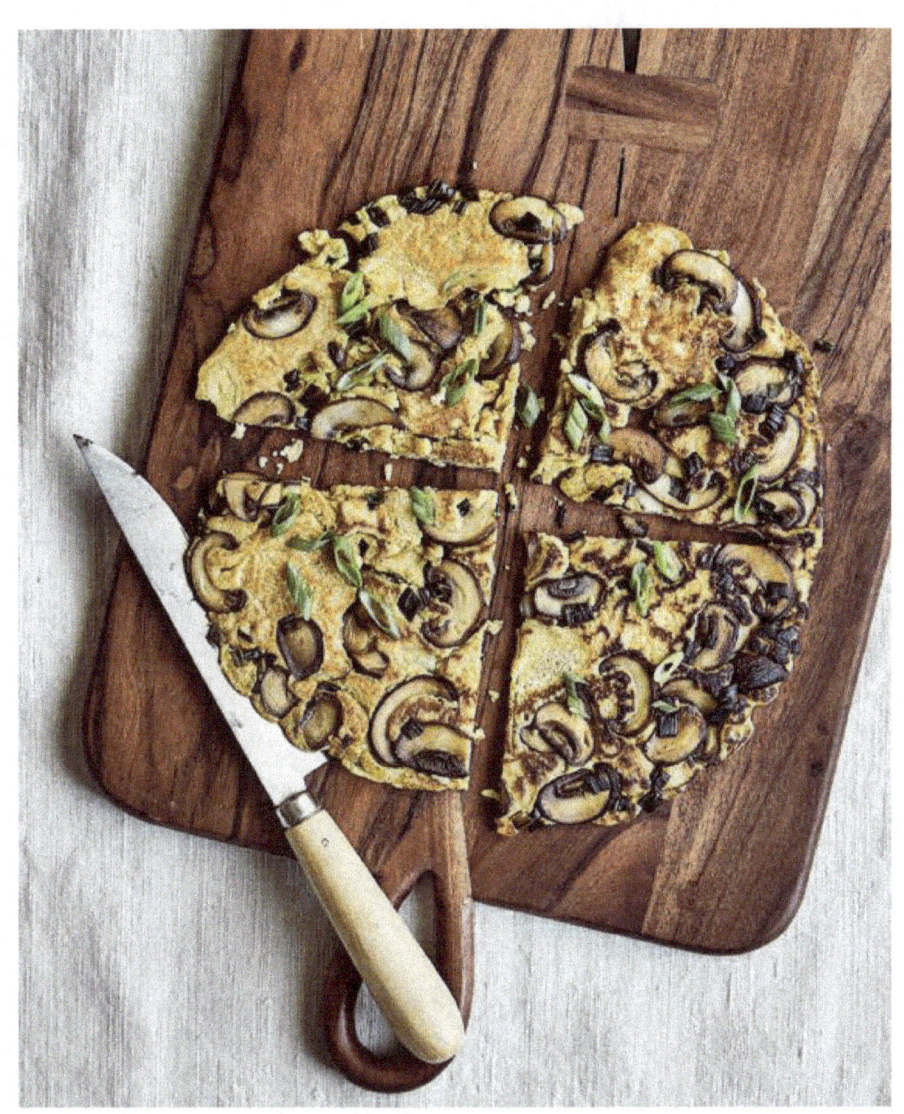

Mushroom and Scallion Chickpea Omelet

PREP TIME: 10 minutes

COOK TIME: 15 minutes

GLUTEN-FREE, NUT-FREE, SOY-FREE

SERVES 4

This is a fantastic omelet base to have in your repertoire. It cooks in minutes and is absolutely delicious with any number of toppings. If you like cheese in your omelet, make the Cheddar-Style Cheese Sauce and add it to the omelet while cooking, or sprinkle on a layer of your favorite store-bought dairy-free cheese shreds.

1 cup chickpea flour

⅓ cup nutritional yeast ½

teaspoon garlic powder

½ teaspoon freshly ground black

pepper ¼ teaspoon baking powder

¼ teaspoon salt

1 cup water

1 tablespoon grapeseed or olive oil

6 white button or cremini mushrooms, stems removed and caps thinly

sliced 2 scallions, both green and white parts, chopped

1. In a medium bowl, whisk together the chickpea flour, nutritional yeast, garlic powder, pepper, baking powder, and salt. Add the water and stir to form a thick but pourable batter. If your batter is very thick or clumpy, add additional water, 1 tablespoon at a time, to loosen it.

2. In a large sauté pan or skillet, heat the oil on medium-high heat. Add the mushrooms and scallions and cook for 5 to 7 minutes, or until the mushrooms are browned.

3. Pour the chickpea batter over the mushroom and scallion mix and gently tilt the pan in a circle to spread the batter evenly over the

bottom. Cook for 3 to 4 minutes, or until the underside of the omelet is lightly browned, then carefully flip the entire omelet over and cook the other side for 2 minutes.

4. Transfer to a plate, cut into 4 portions, and serve.

PER SERVING: Calories: 198; Fat: 5g; Protein: 11g; Carbohydrates: 27g; Fiber: 8g

Smoky Barbecue Tempeh Hash

PREP TIME: 10 minutes

COOK TIME: 20 minutes

GLUTEN-FREE, NUT-FREE, ONE POT

SERVES 3

Breakfast hash is warm and comforting, and it's got all the best components—crispy potatoes, onions, veggies, and protein— plus the smoky sweet taste of barbecue sauce. I like to use tempeh in my hash (Tofurky is a great brand and even has a smoky maple version), but you could use any type of vegan sausage link or patty instead.

3 tablespoons grapeseed or extra-virgin olive oil

3 cups frozen shredded hash browns

½ medium onion, diced

1 green bell pepper, diced

1 red bell pepper, diced

1 (7-ounce) package tempeh, diced

½ cup vegan barbecue sauce

½ cup Cheddar-Style Cheese Sauce or shredded Cheddar-style vegan cheese (optional)

1. In a large sauté pan or skillet with a tight-fitting lid, heat the oil on medium-high heat. Add the hash browns and onion and cook, covered, for 10 minutes, tossing occasionally to keep them from sticking to the bottom of the pan.

2. Add the peppers, then cover and continue cooking for an additional 5 minutes, until the vegetables are tender.

3. Add the tempeh and barbecue sauce to the pan, tossing to coat everything. Cook for 5 minutes more, or until the tempeh is warmed through.

4. Top with the cheese sauce (if using) and serve.

TECHNIQUE TIP: Make this an easy weekday breakfast by chopping your veggies the night before and storing them in an airtight container or resealable bag in the refrigerator until ready to use. In the morning just heat up the pan, toss in your ingredients, and let it cook while you start your day.

STRETCH IT: This is a great recipe to "clean out the fridge" with. Dice up any leftover veggies, like zucchini, celery, and mushrooms, and add them to your hash.

PER SERVING: Calories: 527; Fat: 23g; Protein: 19g; Carbohydrates: 68g; Fiber: 8g

Very Berry Smoothie

PREP TIME: 5 minutes

EASY PREP, GLUTEN-FREE, NO COOK, OIL-FREE, SOY-FREE, SUPERFAST

SERVES 3

I love starting my day with a good serving of fruit. But that can be tricky when I'm rushing to get out the door, which is why smoothies are such a great quick breakfast. Make smoothie prep even faster (and the smoothie even thicker) by using prepackaged frozen fruit. You can even buy "smoothie mix" versions that contain a mix of complementary fruits, which are easier on your budget and take up less space in your freezer.

3 bananas, sliced and frozen

3 cups frozen mixed berries

2 cups unsweetened almond milk

1 cup pomegranate or unsweetened apple juice

Add the bananas, berries, almond milk, and pomegranate juice to a high-speed blender (or a stand blender on the ice crush setting) and blend until smooth.

TECHNIQUE TIP: To make your smoothie thicker and add some probiotics and protein to it, replace 1 cup of almond milk with an equal amount of dairy-free coconut yogurt. Try to choose an unsweetened version to reduce the amount of sugar. I like to use Daiya yogurt alternative, but any brand will work.

VARY IT: This is a great base smoothie recipe that you can adjust to create any number of smoothie combinations like mango-peach-strawberry, strawberry-pineapple, or banana-chocolate-peanut butter.

PER SERVING: Calories: 244; Fat: 2g; Protein: 3g; Carbohydrates: 56g; Fiber: 6g

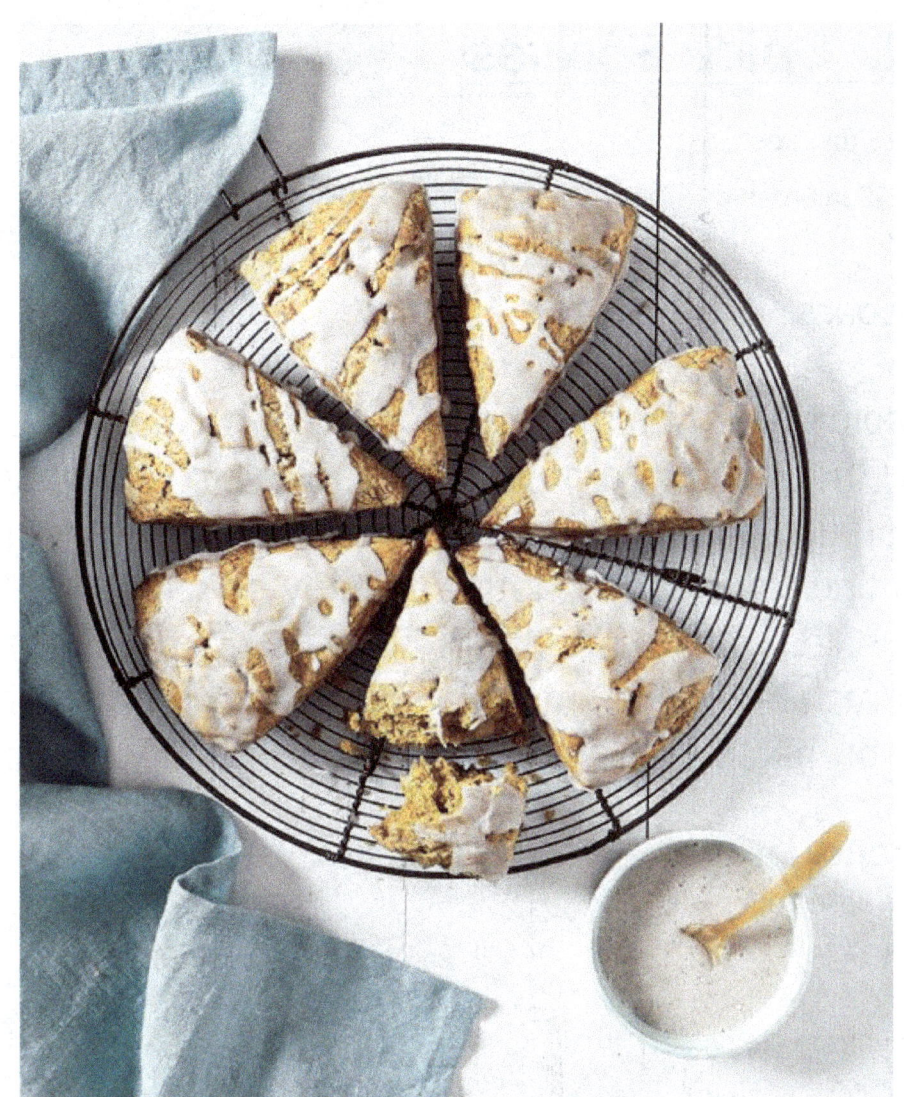

Pumpkin Spice Scones

PREP TIME: 15 minutes

COOK TIME: 15 minutes

NUT-FREE

MAKES 16 SCONES

Fall is absolutely my favorite season, and these scones capture all the warm, aromatic spices of fall in one easy-to-make breakfast staple. The scent of cinnamon, nutmeg, and cloves wafting through the house as they bake reminds me of cooler days, leaves turning bright hues, chunky sweaters, and pumpkin patches. Pumpkin spice scones are the perfect not-too-sweet breakfast treat to go with a strong cup of coffee.

For the scones

4½ cups all-purpose flour

½ cup packed brown sugar

4 teaspoons baking powder

3 teaspoons pumpkin pie spice

1 teaspoon ground cinnamon

½ teaspoon baking soda

1 cup cold vegan butter, cut into 1-inch cubes

1¼ cups canned pumpkin

¾ cup unsweetened soy milk, divided

For the glaze

2 cups confectioners' sugar

3 tablespoons unsweetened soy milk

¼ teaspoon pumpkin pie spice

1. Preheat the oven to 400°F. Line a rimmed baking sheet with parchment paper and set aside.

2. In a large bowl, whisk together the flour, brown sugar, baking

powder, pumpkin pie spice, cinnamon, and baking soda.

3. Using a pastry cutter if you have one (or two knives working in a crisscross cutting motion if you don't), cut the butter into the dry mixture and mix until you have small bits of butter throughout, creating a crumbly texture.

4. Add the pumpkin and ½ cup of soy milk and stir until just combined.

5. Turn out the dough onto a lightly floured surface and knead it with the heels of your hands 8 to 10 times, until it comes together in a ball.

6. Divide the dough in half and shape both halves to form 8-inch circles.

7. Cut the circles into 8 even wedges and place on the prepared baking sheet about 1 inch apart. Brush the wedges with the remaining ¼ cup of soy milk.

8. Bake for 12 to 15 minutes, or until golden. Cool on wire racks for 10 minutes before glazing.

9. To make the glaze: In a small bowl, combine the confectioners' sugar, soy milk, and pumpkin pie spice and whisk until smooth and pourable. Drizzle over the slightly cooled scones and serve.

INGREDIENT TIP: Pumpkin pie spice is a premade spice mix that is available in the spice aisle of almost all supermarkets. It's a combination of ground cinnamon, nutmeg, ginger, allspice, and cloves and is a staple in fall and holiday baking. I like using it because it ta kes up less space than keeping the individual spices on hand—and it's less measuring too. If you can't find pumpkin pie spice in your local grocery store, you can use 2 teaspoons of cinnamon and ½ teaspoon each of nutmeg and ginger for this recipe.

PER SERVING (1 SCONE): Calories: 326; Fat: 12g; Protein: 4g; Carbohydrates: 51g; Fiber: 2g

Mixed Vegetable Tofu Scramble

PREP TIME: 10 minutes

COOK TIME: 15 minutes

NUT-FREE, ONE POT

SERVES 6

This is my go-to tofu scramble recipe. The contents of the scramble may change from week to week based on what's available in my refrigerator, but the result is always delicious. My kids love this scramble with some Cheddar-style cheese melted into it, so when I'm making it for them, I'll include ⅓ cup of vegan cheese shreds, like Daiya. For a spicy southwestern kick, add some black beans and shredded pepper Jack–style vegan cheese.

2 tablespoons grapeseed or extra-virgin olive oil

1 cup sliced cremini mushrooms

1 cup diced zucchini

½ small red onion, diced

½ cup diced red bell pepper

1 cup baby spinach leaves

3 tablespoons low-sodium soy sauce

2 teaspoons minced garlic

2 (14-ounce) blocks extra-firm tofu, drained, pressed, and crumbled

½ cup low-sodium vegetable broth

¼ cup nutritional yeast

½ teaspoon ground turmeric

(optional) Salt

Freshly ground black pepper

1. In a large sauté pan or skillet, heat the oil on medium-high heat. Add the mushrooms, zucchini, onion, and red pepper and cook for 5 minutes, or until the onion is translucent and the mushrooms and

zucchini are soft.

2. Add the spinach, soy sauce, and garlic and cook, stirring, until the spinach is wilted, about 4 minutes.

3. Add the tofu, vegetable broth, nutritional yeast, and turmeric (if using), and stir to combine. Cook for 3 to 4 minutes, or until the broth has been completely absorbed. Season with salt and pepper and serve immediately.

PER SERVING: Calories: 221; Fat: 12g; Protein: 19g; Carbohydrates: 10g; Fiber: 4g

Go Green Smoothie

PREP TIME: 5 minutes

EASY PREP, GLUTEN-FREE, NO COOK, OIL-FREE, SOY-FREE, SUPERFAST

SERVES 3

Don't let the bright green hue of this smoothie fool you. It's full of fruity flavor and is an excellent way to sneak an extra serving of veggies into your day. To give this on-the-go breakfast even more nutritional punch, try adding a scoop of hemp hearts or chia seeds or even some almond butter as you're blending it.

2 bananas

2 cups unsweetened almond milk

2 cups frozen tropical fruit mix (mango and pineapple)

2 cups spinach, fresh or frozen

Add the bananas, almond milk, tropical fruit mix, and spinach to a high-speed blender (or a stand blender on the ice crush setting) and blend until smooth.

PER SERVING: Calories: 159; Fat: 2g; Protein: 3g; Carbohydrates: 34g; Fiber: 4g

Parsley and Chive Pancakes

PREP TIME: 5 minutes

COOK TIME: 15 minutes

EASY PREP, SOY-FREE

SERVES 4

These pancakes are a take on a pancake I used to get at a family-friendly restaurant as a small child. Their kids' menu featured a spaghetti dish that was served with a savory pancake instead of garlic bread, and it was my favorite thing ever. Because I prefer savory over sweet breakfasts, I came up with a version that reminded me of that childhood meal and that made a nice change to our usual pancake mornings.

2 tablespoons hot water
1 tablespoon ground flaxseed
1 cup all-purpose flour
1 tablespoon sugar
1 tablespoon dried parsley
1 tablespoon dried chives
1 teaspoon baking powder
½ teaspoon garlic powder
½ teaspoon onion
powder ¼ teaspoon salt
1 cup unsweetened almond milk
2 tablespoons vegetable oil
Vegan butter, for topping (optional)

1. In a small bowl, combine the hot water and flaxseed. Let it sit for 5 minutes.
2. In a large bowl, combine the flour, sugar, parsley, chives, baking powder, garlic powder, onion powder, and salt.
3. Add the almond milk, vegetable oil, and flaxseed mixture and whisk

to form a batter.

4. Heat a large nonstick skillet over medium-low heat. Working with one pancake at a time, ladle ¼ cup of the pancake batter into the skillet, spreading it into an even circle using the bottom of the measuring cup. Cook for 2 minutes, or until the batter starts to bubble, then crater. Flip and cook for 1 more minute. Repeat with the remaining batter until you have 8 pancakes.

5. Top with a bit of vegan butter (if using) and serve.

PER SERVING: Calories: 209; Fat: 9g; Protein: 4g; Carbohydrates: 29g; Fiber: 2g

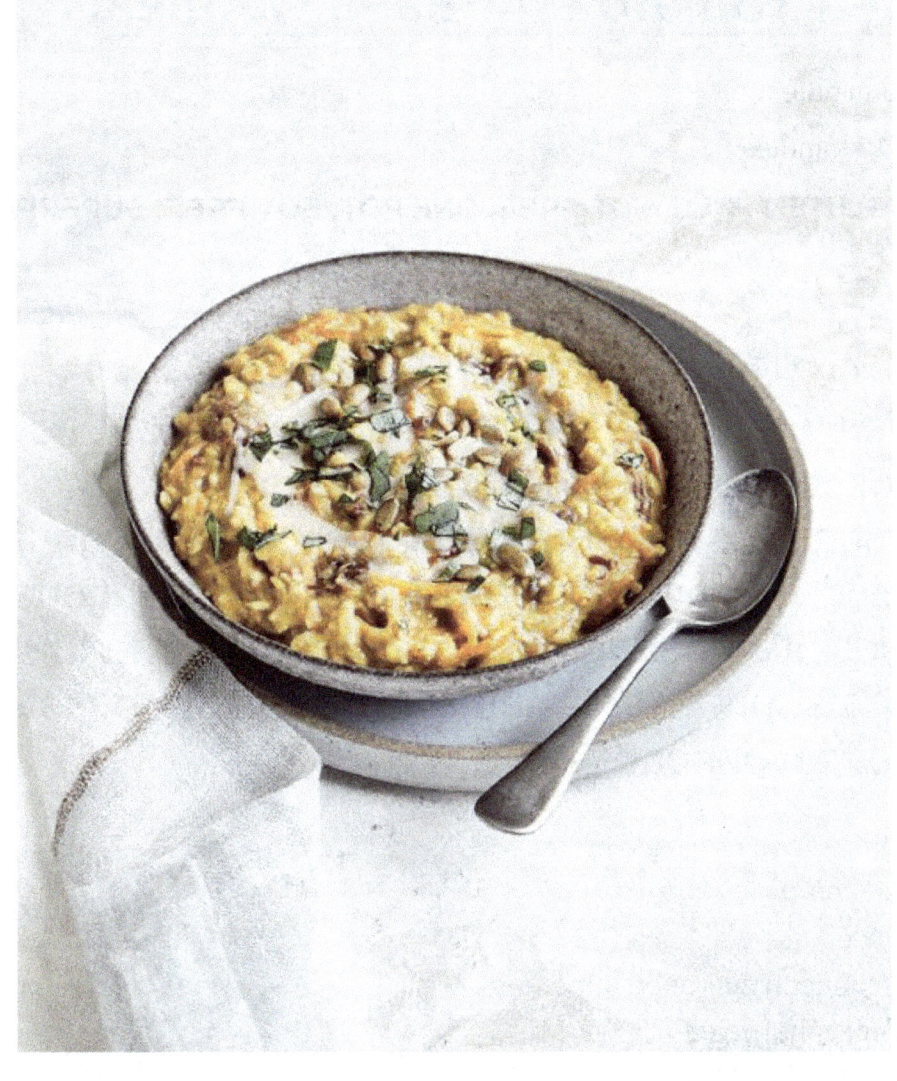

Sun-Dried Tomato and Basil Oatmeal

PREP TIME: 5 minutes

COOK TIME: 10 minutes

EASY PREP, GLUTEN-FREE, NUT-FREE, ONE POT, SOY-FREE, SUPERFAST

SERVES 2

Not what you were expecting, right? Stick with me here for a moment. I was a little skeptical at first too, but now I'm totally hooked. Savory toppings are a great way to shake up a traditionally sweet breakfast dish, and because this recipe includes vitamin powerhouses, like nutritional yeast and veggies, it's good for you too. You can use this base recipe of oats, broth, and nutritional yeast to make any variation of savory oatmeal.

1 tablespoon grapeseed or olive oil

½ cup shredded carrots

½ teaspoon minced garlic

2 tablespoons chopped sun-dried tomatoes

1 tablespoon nutritional yeast

1 tablespoon tahini

1½ teaspoons chopped fresh basil

½ teaspoon apple cider vinegar

¼ teaspoon ground turmeric

2½ cups low-sodium vegetable broth 1 cup rolled oats

Optional toppings: pumpkin seeds, tahini, fresh basil, nutritional yeast

1. In a medium pot, heat the oil on medium-high heat. Add the carrots and garlic and cook until soft, about 3 minutes.

2. Add the sun-dried tomatoes, nutritional yeast, tahini, basil, vinegar, and turmeric and cook for 1 to 2 minutes, until fragrant.

3. Add the vegetable broth and oats and bring to a boil. Immediately reduce the heat to medium and cook, stirring frequently, until the oatmeal reaches your desired consistency. About 5 minutes will get it to thick but creamy (not stiff).

4. Transfer to bowls, add toppings (if using), and serve.

INGREDIENT TIP: If gluten is a concern, check to make sure your oats are certified gluten-free, as cross-contamination sometimes occurs.

PER SERVING: Calories: 310; Fat: 14g; Protein: 10g; Carbohydrates: 38g; Fiber: 7g

3

Salads and Bowls

Tangy Sesame Garden Salad
Spicy Italian Salad with Chickpeas
Chopped Avocado Chickpea Salad with Olives
Dill Pickle Pasta Salad
Caesar Pasta Salad
Buffalo Ranch Pasta Salad
Creamy Broccoli Slaw Salad
Spicy Chickpea Bowls
Tofu Shawarma Bowls with Pearl Couscous
Veggie Fajita Bowls
Crispy Teriyaki Tofu Vermicelli Bowls
Tempeh Bulgogi Rice Bowls
Watermelon Poke Bowls
Spicy Peanut Tofu Mango Bowls
Veggie Bibimbap
Greek Veggie Bowls with Hummus

Tangy Sesame Garden Salad

PREP TIME: 10 minutes

GLUTEN-FREE, NO COOK, SUPERFAST

SERVES 4

This is my always-on-repeat summer salad. It hits all the right notes: it's light, fresh, crispy, tangy, and so satisfying. And it's totally customizable by swapping some lettuce for napa cabbage; adding bell peppers, celery, or carrots; swapping the mandarins for strawberries . . . the possibilities are endless. For extra texture and flavor, add some cooked store-bought vegan chick'n strips.

For the dressing

½ cup rice vinegar

¼ cup plus 2 tablespoons sesame oil

¼ cup sugar

2 tablespoons vegetable oil

3 teaspoons tamari

For the salad

1 head iceberg lettuce, chopped

1 seedless cucumber, chopped

2 (10-ounce) cans mandarin orange slices, drained

8 ounces sugar snap peas, halved

½ cup sliced or slivered almonds

¼ cup sliced radishes (5 or 6 large ones)

1. To make the dressing: In a jar with a tight-fitting lid, combine the rice vinegar, sesame oil, sugar, vegetable oil, and tamari. Shake well to combine.

2. To make the salad: In a large bowl, combine the lettuce, cucumber, mandarin oranges, snap peas, almonds, and radishes. Toss with

dressing to taste and serve.

PER SERVING: Calories: 480; Fat: 34g; Protein: 8g; Carbohydrates: 39g; Fiber: 7g

Spicy Italian Salad with Chickpeas

PREP TIME: 20 minutes

GLUTEN-FREE, NO COOK, NUT-FREE, SOY-FREE

SERVES 6

This is the perfect picnic or potluck salad, and it takes just minutes to make. It gets its "spicy" moniker from the addition of red pepper flakes in the dressing and from the heat of both red onion and pepperoncini.

For the dressing
½ cup grapeseed or extra-virgin olive oil 3 tablespoons red or white wine vinegar 1 teaspoon Dijon mustard

1 teaspoon sugar

½ teaspoon Italian seasoning

¼ teaspoon salt

¼ teaspoon freshly ground black pepper

¼ teaspoon red pepper flakes

For the salad
1 medium head iceberg lettuce, torn or chopped

1 (5-ounce) package spring mix salad greens

2 (15-ounce) cans chickpeas, drained and rinsed

2 cups halved cherry tomatoes

¼ red onion, thinly sliced

½ cup pitted, sliced black olives

6 to 8 whole pepperoncini, for topping

1. To make the dressing: In a small bowl, whisk together the oil, vinegar, mustard, sugar, Italian seasoning, salt, black pepper, and red pepper flakes and whisk to combine.
2. To make the salad: In a large bowl, combine the lettuce and salad

greens, chickpeas, tomatoes, onion, and olives. Toss
with the dressing and top with pepperoncini to serve.

SMART SHOPPING: If you're like me and despise prepping lettuce, swap the head of lettuce for 2
(6-ounce) bags of prewashed, chopped lettuce and turn this into a 15-minute meal.

PER SERVING: Calories: 334; Fat: 22g; Protein: 9g; Carbohydrates: 28g; Fiber: 8g

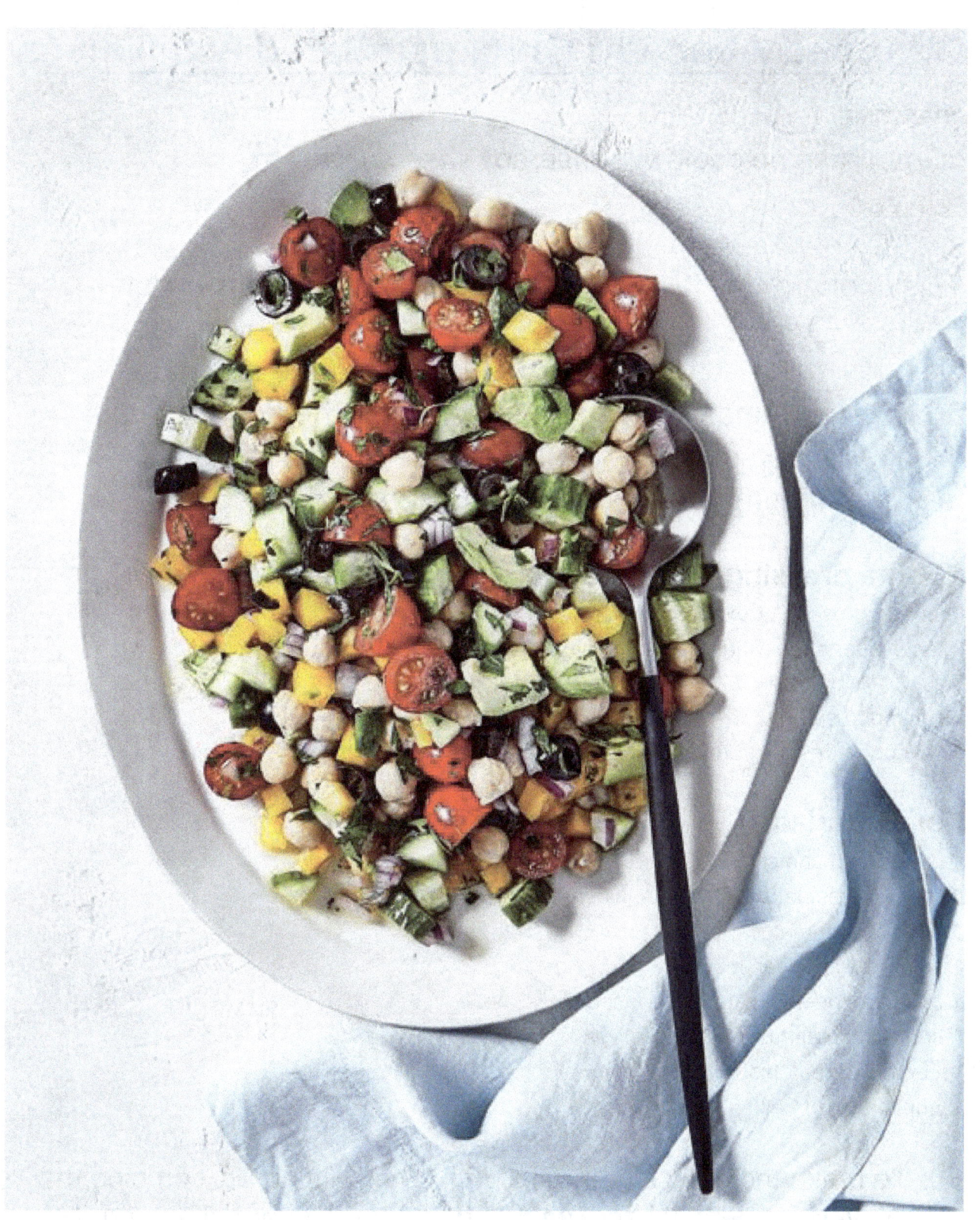

Chopped Avocado Chickpea Salad with Olives

PREP TIME: 15 minutes

GLUTEN-FREE, NO COOK, NUT-FREE, SOY-FREE, SUPERFAST

SERVES 6

This is one of my favorite salads. It's my take on a Middle Eastern chopped salad I grew up eating. The chickpeas give this salad added protein and fiber and the avocado adds a creaminess that pairs so well with the snappy bite from the onion and parsley. I like to serve this salad with falafel and hummus for a Middle Eastern–style feast.

For the dressing

¼ cup grapeseed or extra-virgin olive oil

3 tablespoons red wine or apple cider vinegar

Juice of ½ lemon

¼ teaspoon salt

¼ teaspoon freshly ground black pepper

For the salad

1 (15-ounce) can chickpeas, drained and rinsed

2 medium seedless cucumbers, diced

1 pint grape tomatoes, halved

1 yellow bell pepper, diced

1 avocado, peeled, pitted, and diced

1 cup sliced kalamata or black olives

½ cup diced red onion

½ cup chopped fresh flat-leaf parsley

1. To make the dressing: In a jar with a tight-fitting lid, combine the oil, vinegar, lemon juice, salt, and pepper. Cover tightly and shake to combine.

2. To make the salad: In a large bowl, combine the chickpeas,

cucumbers, tomatoes, bell pepper, avocado, olives, red onion, and parsley. Add the dressing, toss to combine, and serve.

PER SERVING: Calories: 247; Fat: 17g; Protein: 6g; Carbohydrates: 22g; Fiber: 7g

Dill Pickle Pasta Salad

PREP TIME: 15 minutes

COOK TIME: 15 minutes

NUT-FREE

SERVES 8

I love dill pickles and I'll put them in just about anything, so it's no surprise that this is one of my favorite pasta dishes. This salad uses both diced pickles in the salad and pickle juice in the dressing, giving it a one-two briny pickle punch. This pasta salad is delicious when first made but also gets better as it chills, making it a great make-ahead party dish.

For the salad

1 (16-ounce) box elbow macaroni

3 celery stalks, diced

¾ cup diced kosher dill

pickles ½ red onion, diced

½ red bell pepper, diced

2 tablespoons chopped fresh dill or 1 tablespoon dried dill

For the dressing

1 cup Vegan Mayonnaise or store-bought

3 tablespoons dill pickle juice

2 tablespoons sugar

½ teaspoon freshly ground black

pepper ¼ teaspoon salt

1. Bring a large pot of water to a boil and cook the macaroni according to package directions.

2. To make the dressing: While the pasta is cooking, in a small bowl, combine the mayonnaise, pickle juice, sugar, pepper, and salt and whisk until combined. Set aside.

3. Drain and rinse the pasta under cold running water, drain well, and place in a large bowl.

4. Add the celery, pickles, red onion, bell pepper, and dill to the pasta. Add the dressing, toss to combine, and serve.

INGREDIENT TIP: Kosher dill pickles were named for their preparation by classic kosher-style New York delis, and not necessarily under the supervision of a rabbi (as is the custom with most kosher products). A kosher dill pickle is similar to a regular dill pickle, but with a few subtle changes that make it unique. Kosher dills are brined with generous amounts of garlic and dill in a natural salt brine, and are brined longer, making them sourer than regular dills.

PER SERVING: Calories: 356; Fat: 15g; Protein: 8g; Carbohydrates: 48g; Fiber: 3g

Caesar Pasta Salad

PREP TIME: 10 minutes

COOK TIME: 10 minutes

NUT-FREE

SERVES 6

Caesar salad lovers, rejoice! This dressing is so creamy, tangy, and delicious it's almost indistinguishable from its non-vegan counterpart. This salad comes together in the time it takes to boil pasta and is even better with some quick pan-fried tofu or vegan bacon.

For the salad

1 (16-ounce) box whole-wheat rotini pasta

1 (10-ounce) bag chopped romaine lettuce

1 seedless cucumber, halved and sliced

1 pint cherry tomatoes, halved

1 cup store-bought vegan croutons (optional)

For the dressing

½ cup Vegan Mayonnaise or store-bought 2 tablespoons freshly squeezed lemon juice 2 tablespoons nutritional yeast

2 tablespoons capers, drained

1 tablespoon Dijon mustard

1 tablespoon low-sodium soy sauce

1 tablespoon extra-virgin olive oil

1 tablespoon maple syrup

½ teaspoon minced garlic

¼ teaspoon white vinegar

1. Bring a large pot of water to a boil and cook the pasta according to package directions.

2. To make the dressing: While the pasta is cooking, in a blender, combine the mayonnaise, lemon juice, nutritional yeast, capers, Dijon mustard, soy sauce, olive oil, maple syrup, garlic, and vinegar, and process until creamy.

3. Drain and rinse the pasta under cold running water and drain well.

4. In a large bowl, combine the lettuce, cucumber, and tomatoes. Add the pasta and ½ cup of the dressing. Toss to combine and top with the croutons (if using) to serve.

STRETCH IT: This recipe makes a full cup of dressing, but only half is needed for this dish. Store the remaining dressing in the refrigerator for up to 5 days and use it on another dish later in the week.

PER SERVING: Calories: 352; Fat: 8g; Protein: 13g; Carbohydrates: 62g; Fiber: 10g

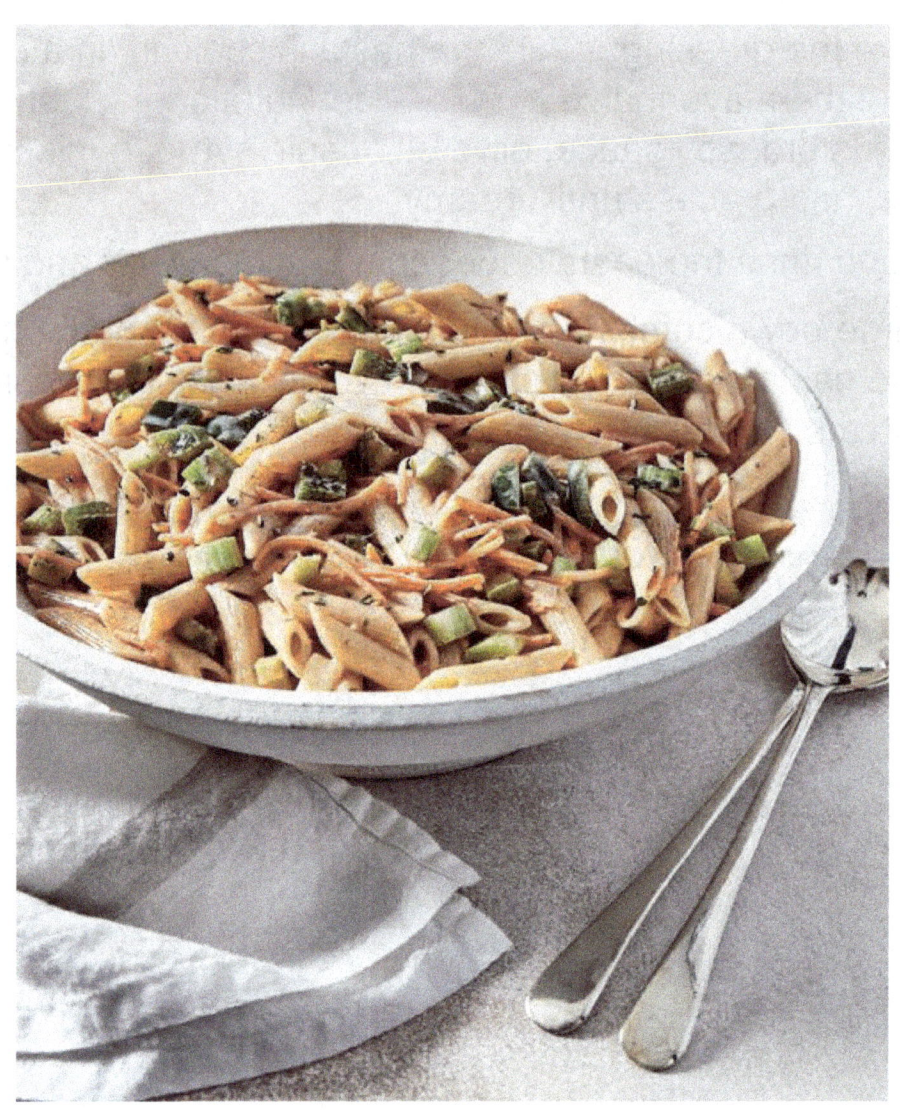

Buffalo Ranch Pasta Salad

PREP TIME: 10 minutes

COOK TIME: 15 minutes

NUT-FREE

SERVES 6

My husband was a huge wing fan in his pre-vegan days, and buffalo wings with a really good ranch dip were always his favorite. I created this pasta salad to switch up the classic pasta salad and mimic the flavors of wing night. Fiery-hot buffalo sauce followed by the cooling sensation of ranch makes this a delicious game day or backyard gathering dish.

For the salad

1 (16-ounce) box penne pasta

2 carrots, shredded

2 celery stalks, diced

1 green bell pepper, diced

½ cup Louisiana-style hot sauce (I prefer Frank's RedHot)

For the dressing

1½ cups Vegan Mayonnaise or store-bought

½ cup unsweetened soy milk

1½ teaspoons white or apple cider vinegar

1½ teaspoons dried parsley

1 teaspoon minced garlic

1 teaspoon dried dill

1 teaspoon onion powder

¼ teaspoon salt

¼ teaspoon freshly ground black pepper

1. Bring a large pot of water to a boil and cook the pasta according to package directions.

2. To make the dressing: While the pasta is cooking, in a medium bowl, combine the mayonnaise, soy milk, vinegar, parsley, garlic, dill, onion powder, salt, and pepper. Whisk until well mixed.

3. In a large bowl, combine the carrots, celery, and bell pepper.

4. Drain the pasta, rinse under cold running water, and drain well. Add the cooked pasta, hot sauce, and ¾ cup of the dressing to the vegetables. Toss to combine and serve.

STRETCH IT: This recipe makes almost 2 cups of ranch dressing. Store the remaining dressing in an airtight container in the refrigerator for up to a week. If you don't feel like making your own ranch dressing, any vegan store-bought brand will work just as well.

PER SERVING: Calories: 425; Fat: 15g; Protein: 11g; Carbohydrates: 61g; Fiber: 4g

Creamy Broccoli Slaw Salad

PREP TIME: 20 minutes

GLUTEN-FREE, NO COOK

SERVES 6

If you're not a raw broccoli fan, this salad will change your mind. It's creamy, tangy, crunchy, and absolutely delicious. The trick to this salad is to cut your broccoli florets small enough so that they are bite-size. I use precut bagged broccoli florets and trim the larger ones. If you're able to find vegan blue cheese, pick some up and crumble it on top of this salad for an extra-indulgent treat.

For the dressing

¾ cup unsweetened dairy-free yogurt (I prefer Daiya) ⅓ cup Vegan Mayonnaise or store-bought

2 tablespoons maple syrup or agave nectar

1½ tablespoons apple cider vinegar

¼ teaspoon salt

For the salad

4 cups broccoli florets, cut small (about 2 [12-ounce] bags)

2 small Gala apples, diced

1 cup shredded carrots

1 cup slivered or sliced almonds

½ cup dried cranberries

¼ cup diced red onion

1. To make the dressing: In a medium bowl whisk together the yogurt, mayonnaise, maple syrup, vinegar, and salt.
2. To make the salad: In a large salad bowl, combine the broccoli florets, apples, carrots, almonds, cranberries, and onion. Toss with the dressing and serve.

PER SERVING: Calories: 303; Fat: 17g; Protein: 7g; Carbohydrates: 34g; Fiber: 7g

Spicy Chickpea Bowls

PREP TIME: 10 minutes

COOK TIME: 20 minutes

NUT-FREE, SOY-FREE

SERVES 6

In this hearty bowl, the chickpeas are wonderfully spiced, with heat from the chili powder and cumin and the savory-sweetness of cinnamon. If you want to keep this bowl low carb, swap the rice for chopped romaine lettuce.

For the rice

4 cups low-sodium vegetable broth or water

2 cups basmati rice, rinsed

For the spicy chickpeas

2 tablespoons grapeseed or extra-virgin olive oil

½ medium onion, diced

1 tablespoon ground cumin

1 tablespoon chili powder

½ teaspoon ground turmeric

½ teaspoon salt

¼ teaspoon ground cinnamon

1 (28-ounce) can chickpeas, drained and rinsed

1 (28-ounce) can diced tomatoes

For the bowls

4 whole-wheat pitas

1 seedless cucumber

2 lemons

1 cup hummus

6 tablespoons tahini, for topping

1. To make the rice: In a medium pot, bring the vegetable broth to a boil. Add the rice, stir, and reduce the heat to low. Cover and cook for 15minutes.

2. While the rice is cooking, in a large sauté pan or skillet, heat the oil on medium-high heat. Add the onion and cook for 5 minutes, or until just translucent.

3. Add the cumin, chili powder, turmeric, salt, and cinnamon and stir until the onions are just coated. Add the chickpeas and tomatoes and their juices and simmer for 15 minutes, until the flavors meld.

4. While the chickpeas and rice are cooking, cut the pitas into wedges, dice the cucumber, and quarter the lemons lengthwise.

5. In each bowl, place ½ cup of rice. Top with chickpeas, cucumber, hummus, and pita. Squeeze a lemon wedge over each bowl, drizzle each with 1 tablespoon of tahini, and serve.

MAKE IT AHEAD: Make the rice ahead of time or use any leftover rice (or quinoa) you may have to form the base of this bowl.

PER SERVING: Calories: 728; Fat: 22g; Protein: 24g; Carbohydrates: 115g; Fiber: 17g

Tofu Shawarma Bowls with Pearl Couscous

PREP TIME: 15 minutes

COOK TIME: 15 minutes

NUT-FREE

SERVES 4

This dish is all about the seasoning. We capture the warm, fragrant spices of shawarma mix, a Middle Eastern seasoning blend, in a quick and easy paste that we use to baste the tofu. I like serving this bowl on pearl couscous, but any grain you have on hand will do. Pearl couscous cooks in just 10 minutes, so you can make it while you prep the rest of the meal.

For the couscous

1¼ cups water

1 cup dry pearl or Israeli couscous

For the dressing

⅓ cup tahini

⅓ cup water

¼ cup plus 1 tablespoon freshly squeezed lemon

juice 2 garlic cloves, peeled

¾ teaspoon salt

For the tofu shawarma

3 tablespoons grapeseed or extra-virgin olive oil, divided

½ teaspoon ground coriander

½ teaspoon ground cumin ¼

teaspoon ground cinnamon ¼

teaspoon garlic powder

¼ teaspoon chili powder ¼

teaspoon ground ginger

1 (14-ounce) block extra-firm tofu, drained, patted dry, and cut into 1-inch

cubes 1 seedless cucumber, diced

½ pint grape tomatoes, halved

½ cup store-bought sliced pickled turnips or beets (optional)

1. To make the couscous: In a small pot, combine the water and couscous. Bring to a boil, then reduce the heat to low. Cover and simmer for 10 minutes. Fluff with a fork.

2. To make the dressing: In a small food processor or blender, combine the tahini, water, lemon juice, garlic, and salt and process until combined. Set aside.

3. In a medium bowl, combine 1 tablespoon of oil, coriander, cumin, cinnamon, garlic powder, chili powder, and ginger. Add the tofu and toss to coat.

4. In a large sauté pan or skillet, heat the remaining 2 tablespoons of oil over medium-high heat. Add the coated tofu to the skillet and cook, tossing occasionally, until the tofu is crispy on all sides, about 10 minutes.

5. Place about ⅓ cup of couscous in each bowl. Divide the tofu, cucumber, and tomatoes evenly between the bowls. Top with a few pickled turnips (if using), drizzle with the dressing, and serve.

MAKE IT AHEAD: Both the couscous and the tofu can be made ahead of time to keep this dish even easier to assemble. Prepare both and keep in airtight containers in the refrigerator, then gently warm in the microwave just before serving.

PER SERVING: Calories: 492; Fat: 27g; Protein: 20g; Carbohydrates: 48g; Fiber: 6g

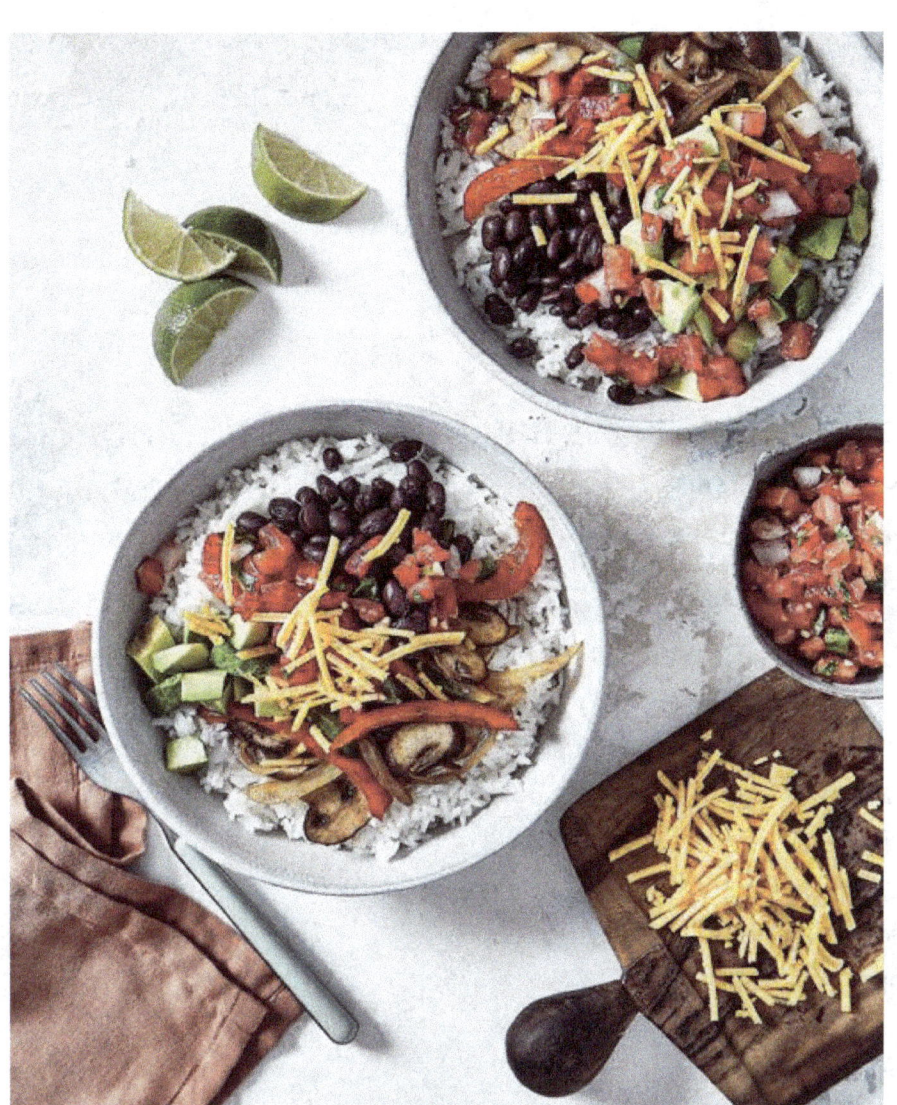

Veggie Fajita Bowls

PREP TIME: 15 minutes

COOK TIME: 15 minutes

GLUTEN-FREE, NUT-FREE, SOY-FREE

SERVES 4

These bowls offer all the flavors of fajitas without the messiness of wraps. I like to use basmati (or any long-grain) rice in this dish, and I cook the rice in vegetable broth instead of water to give it some flavor. If you want to add a dressing to this bowl, I highly recommend the vegan ranch dressing recipe from my Buffalo Ranch Pasta Salad.

2 cups low-sodium vegetable broth

1 cup basmati rice, rinsed

2 tablespoons grapeseed or extra-virgin olive oil

1 medium onion, cut into half moons

1 red bell pepper, cut into strips

1 green bell pepper, cut into strips

1 cup sliced cremini mushrooms

1½ tablespoons chili powder

1 (15-ounce) can black beans, drained and rinsed

1 avocado, peeled, pitted, and diced

1 cup store-bought salsa

1 cup shredded Cheddar- or pepper Jack–style vegan cheese (I prefer Daiya)

1 lime, quartered

1. In a small pot, combine the vegetable broth and rice. Bring to a boil, then reduce the heat to low. Cover and cook for 15 minutes. Remove from the heat and fluff with a fork.

2. While the rice is cooking, in a large sauté pan or skillet, heat the oil on medium-high heat until shimmering. Add the onion, peppers, mushrooms, and chili powder and toss to coat. Cook until soft, about

10 minutes.

3. Divide the rice evenly into bowls. Top with the cooked vegetables, black beans, avocado, salsa, and cheese. Serve with a slice of lime.

TECHNIQUE TIP: To slice onions into half moons, trim the ends off the onion and cut it in half lengthwise to form two semi-circles. Lay each semi-circle flat and thinly slice crosswise into strips, and voilà: half moons!

PER SERVING: Calories: 535; Fat: 19g; Protein: 13g; Carbohydrates: 83g; Fiber: 15g

Crispy Teriyaki Tofu Vermicelli Bowls

PREP TIME: 15 minutes

COOK TIME: 15 minutes

SERVES 3

My kids and I love getting tofu teriyaki from the food court at the mall. But the fast food version isn't the healthiest, and it's not always a convenient option. I created this homemade version to satisfy our take-out cravings, while balancing the amount of salt and fat in the dish. What I also love about this recipe is how customizable it is. This is the perfect dish to play "clean out the fridge" with at the end of a week.

For the base

1 (14-ounce) package rice vermicelli noodles

2 tablespoons grapeseed or extra-virgin olive oil

1 (14-ounce) block extra-firm tofu, drained, patted dry, and cut into cubes

3 tablespoons cornstarch

For the sauce

¼ cup low-sodium soy sauce

3 tablespoons packed brown sugar

2 tablespoons grapeseed or extra-virgin olive oil

1 tablespoon maple syrup

½ teaspoon grated ginger

¼ teaspoon garlic powder

For the bowls

1 seedless cucumber, cut into half moons

2 cups romaine or iceberg lettuce, chopped

⅓ cup chopped peanuts

1. Bring a large pot of water to a boil and cook the vermicelli noodles

according to package directions. Drain and set aside.

2. In a large sauté pan or skillet, heat the oil over medium-high heat. In a small bowl, toss the tofu with the cornstarch to coat. Add the tofu to the hot pan and cook, tossing occasionally, until crispy and golden on all sides, about 10 minutes.

3. To make the sauce: While the tofu is cooking, in a small bowl, combine the soy sauce, brown sugar, oil, maple syrup, ginger, and garlic powder.

4. Once the tofu is golden, add ½ cup of the sauce to the pan and toss the tofu to coat. Cook for 2 minutes, or until the sauce thickens and is sticky. Remove from the heat.

5. To make the bowls: Divide the cooked, drained noodles evenly into bowls. Top with the tofu, cucumber, lettuce, and peanuts. Drizzle the remaining sauce over the bowls and serve.

SMART SHOPPING: Speed up this recipe by using a store-bought teriyaki sauce instead of homemade. Try to choose a low-sodium version to reduce the amount of salt in your dish.

STRETCH IT: This recipe makes double the amount of teriyaki sauce you'll need for the recipe. Use the remaining sauce to drizzle over your bowl or keep it in the refrigerator in an airtight container for up to a week.

PER SERVING: Calories: 985; Fat: 36g; Protein: 29g; Carbohydrates: 142g; Fiber: 7g

Tempeh Bulgogi Rice Bowls

PREP TIME: 10 minutes

COOK TIME: 15 minutes

NUT-FREE

SERVES 4

The first place my now-husband and I moved into was a condo building with a retail shopping level on the ground floor. One of those retail stores was a Korean barbecue restaurant, and it quickly became a favorite hangout. In my pre-vegan days, I loved beef bulgogi, and now I've created my own vegan version to replicate that savory, sweet spicy flavor.

For the bowls

2 cups water

1 cup basmati rice, rinsed

2 tablespoons grapeseed or extra-virgin olive oil

½ medium onion, thinly sliced

4 ounces green beans

1 (7-ounce) package tempeh, diced or crumbled

Sesame seeds, for garnish (optional)

Sriracha, for garnish (optional)

For the bulgogi sauce

¾ cup low-sodium soy sauce

¾ cup brown sugar

¾ cup no-added-sugar apple juice

3 scallions, both white and green parts, finely chopped

1 tablespoon minced garlic

1 tablespoon grated ginger

1 tablespoon sesame oil

1. In a small pot, combine the water and rice and bring to a boil.

Immediately reduce the heat to low, stir, cover, and cook for 15 minutes. Remove from the heat and fluff with a fork.

2. To make the bulgogi sauce: While the rice is cooking, in a small saucepan, combine the soy sauce, brown sugar, and apple juice. Warm over low heat just until the sugar dissolves. Remove from the heat and stir in the scallions, garlic, ginger, and sesame oil. Set aside.

3. In a large sauté pan or skillet, heat the grapeseed oil over medium-high heat. Add the onion and green beans and cook until the onion is translucent, about 5 minutes.

4. Add the tempeh and bulgogi sauce to the skillet and cook for about 10 minutes, until the tempeh is soft and the sauce has reduced slightly.

5. Add ½ cup of rice to each bowl, top with tempeh and onions, and drizzle with extra sauce. Sprinkle the sesame seeds and sriracha (if using) on top and serve.

INGREDIENT TIP: Bulgogi sauce is a Korean marinade traditionally used on beef. It is also often referred to simply as Korean barbecue marinade or sauce. It has spicy notes from the garlic and ginger, and sweetness from brown sugar and apple or pear juice, and pairs well with any faux beef. It is available at many mainstream grocery stores in the Asian or international foods aisle. Swap the homemade version here for store-bought to make this dish even faster.

PER SERVING: Calories: 518; Fat: 16g; Protein: 18g; Carbohydrates: 79g; Fiber: 3g

Watermelon Poke Bowls

PREP TIME: 25 minutes

COOK TIME: 5 minutes

GLUTEN-FREE, NUT-FREE

SERVES 4

A poke bowl is typically served with raw, diced fish like salmon or tuna. Here, watermelon brings a vegan twist. Poke bowls are also often served with rice, which you can add to this recipe if you like.

For the dressing

½ cup Vegan Mayonnaise or store-
bought 2 tablespoons rice vinegar

2 tablespoons low-sodium soy sauce

2 tablespoons grated ginger

2 teaspoons sugar

2 teaspoons sesame oil

4 teaspoons sesame seeds

For the watermelon poke

1 cup frozen shelled edamame

4 cups packed baby spinach

6 cups diced seedless watermelon (about ¼ watermelon)

1 seedless cucumber, sliced into half moons

1 avocado, peeled, pitted, and diced

1 tablespoon chopped pickled jalapeño

4 tablespoons black sesame seeds, for garnish (optional)

1. To make the dressing: In a small bowl, combine the mayonnaise, rice vinegar, soy sauce, ginger, sugar, and sesame oil. Whisk until smooth. Stir in the sesame seeds.

2. Fill a small saucepan halfway with water and bring to a boil. Cook the

edamame for 2 minutes, then drain and rinse under cold water until cool. Pat dry.

3. Divide the spinach evenly between 4 bowls. Add the watermelon, cucumber, avocado, and edamame. Top with the jalapeño and sprinkle with black sesame seeds (if using). Drizzle with the dressing and serve.

MAKE IT AHEAD: The dressing for this recipe is fantastic on all sorts of salads and lasts in the refrigerator for up to a week. Try making it a day or two in advance and storing it in an airtight container until needed.

PER SERVING: Calories: 342; Fat: 25g; Protein: 10g; Carbohydrates: 24g; Fiber: 6g

Spicy Peanut Tofu Mango Bowls

PREP TIME: 10 minutes

COOK TIME: 15 minutes

SERVES 4

I've made this dish so many times I could practically do it in my sleep. I blame the sauce. It's rich, creamy, spicy, and sweet —perfect with tofu, juicy mango, and crisp red peppers. It also makes a fantastic dip for rice paper rolls, a dressing (thinned out with a bit of oil or coconut milk), or a glaze. It keeps in the refrigerator for 4 to 5 days.

For the bowls

7 ounces wide rice noodles

1 tablespoon grapeseed or extra-virgin olive oil

2 (14-ounce) blocks extra-firm tofu, drained, pressed, and cut into 1-inch cubes

2 tablespoons cornstarch

2 cups diced mango (fresh or frozen, thawed)

1 red bell pepper, cut into strips

½ cup chopped fresh flat-leaf parsley or cilantro, for

garnish ¼ cup crushed peanuts, for garnish

For the sauce

½ cup sweet Thai chili sauce

¼ cup low-sodium soy sauce

3 tablespoons creamy peanut

butter Juice of 1 lime

1 tablespoon sugar

2 teaspoons minced garlic

1. Bring a large pot of water to a boil, add the noodles, and cook according to package directions. Drain and rinse under cold water to keep from sticking.

2. To make the sauce: In a medium bowl, combine the chili sauce, soy sauce, peanut butter, lime juice, sugar, and garlic. Whisk until well combined.

3. In a large sauté pan or skillet, heat the oil on medium-high heat. Meanwhile, in a large bowl, combine the tofu and cornstarch and toss to coat. Add the tofu to the hot skillet and cook for about 10 minutes, until crispy and golden on all sides.

4. Add the sauce to the skillet and simmer for 2 to 3 minutes, or until the sauce thickens slightly.

5. Divide the cooked rice noodles into bowls. Top with the tofu and sauce. Add the mango and red pepper. Garnish with parsley and peanuts and serve.

PER SERVING: Calories: 730; Fat: 25g; Protein: 32g; Carbohydrates: 87g; Fiber: 7g

Veggie Bibimbap

PREP TIME: 10 minutes

COOK TIME: 15 minutes

NUT-FREE

SERVES 4

Bibimbap is a Korean dish that means "mixed rice." It usually consists of rice, vegetables, meat or tofu, and an egg and is served with an incredibly flavorful red pepper paste called gochujang. Traditionally, each component is cooked separately and artfully laid out on top of the rice, but in the interest of keeping this dish under the 30-minute mark, I cook all the vegetables together, stir-fry style.

2 cups water

1 cup basmati rice, rinsed

2 tablespoons sesame oil, divided

1 (14-ounce) block extra-firm tofu, drained, pressed, and cut into ½-inch-thick strips

4 cups packed baby spinach

2 cups zucchini, thinly sliced into half moons

8 ounces cremini mushrooms, stems removed and caps sliced

1 cup shredded carrots

1 cup bean sprouts

Gochujang or sriracha

Hoisin sauce

1. In a small pot, combine the water and rice and bring to a boil. Immediately reduce the heat to low, stir, cover, and cook for 15 minutes. Remove from the heat and fluff with a fork.

2. Meanwhile, in a large sauté pan or skillet, heat 1 tablespoon of sesame oil on medium-high heat. Add the tofu and cook, turning once, until golden, about 7 minutes. Remove from the pan and set aside.

3. Add the remaining 1 tablespoon of sesame oil to the pan and add the spinach, zucchini, mushrooms, and carrots. Cook for 5 to 7 minutes, or until the mushrooms and zucchini are softened and the spinach is wilted. Remove from the heat and stir in the bean sprouts.

4. Add ½ cup of rice to each bowl. Top with the mixed vegetables, a dollop of gochujang sauce, and 2 or 3 drops of hoisin sauce. Mix to combine and serve.

VARY IT: Give this dish even more meaty flavor by adding the tempeh beef from the Tempeh Bulgogi Rice Bowl.

PER SERVING: Calories: 376; Fat: 13g; Protein: 18g; Carbohydrates: 49g; Fiber: 4g

Greek Veggie Bowls with Hummus

PREP TIME: 10 minutes

COOK TIME: 20 minutes

GLUTEN-FREE, NUT-FREE, SOY-FREE

SERVES 4

This is a hearty, satisfying weekday lunch or dinner bowl that is easy to prepare. I like to prep each component at the beginning of the week to store in the refrigerator until I'm ready to eat, then all I have to do is toss everything in a bowl and go. If you do make this in advance, keep the salad and the dressing separate until you're ready to serve so your veggies don't get soggy.

For the bowls

2 cups water

1 cup quinoa

3 cups prewashed, bagged chopped kale

1 pint cherry tomatoes, halved

½ seedless cucumber, sliced into half moons 1 red bell pepper, diced

½ cup diced red onion

1 cup hummus

12 pitted kalamata olives

For the dressing

⅓ cup grapeseed or extra-virgin olive oil 3 tablespoons apple cider vinegar

1 tablespoon freshly squeezed lemon juice

2 teaspoons minced garlic

1 teaspoon dried oregano

¾ teaspoon salt

½ teaspoon Dijon mustard

½ teaspoon freshly ground black pepper

1. In a small saucepan, bring the water to a boil. Add the quinoa, reduce the heat to low, cover, and cook for 15 minutes. Remove from the heat and let stand for 5 minutes. Fluff with a fork and set aside.

2. To make the dressing: While the quinoa is cooking, in a glass jar with a tight-fitting lid, combine the oil, vinegar, lemon juice, garlic, oregano, salt, mustard, and pepper. Shake well until combined.

3. In a large bowl, combine the kale, tomatoes, cucumber, red bell pepper, and onion. Toss with the dressing.

4. Spoon 1 cup of quinoa into each bowl. Top with the veggies, hummus, and olives and serve.

VARY IT: Add some extra protein to this dish by including the tofu shawarma from the Tofu Shawarma Bowls with Pearl Couscous. The warm, fragrant spices in the tofu pair beautifully with the tangy Greek salad and creamy hummus.

PER SERVING: Calories: 557; Fat: 34g; Protein: 11g; Carbohydrates: 52g; Fiber: 8g

4

Handhelds

Cheesy Summer Squash Flatbreads

Seven-Layer Burritos

Crab Cake Burgers

Veggie Supreme Garlic Bread Pizza

Cashew Curry Tofu Pita Pockets

Tofu-Lettuce-Tomato-Avocado Sandwich

Spinach and Mushroom Baguettes with Garlic-Herb Cream Cheese

Tofu Fish Tacos

Kung Pao Tempeh Lettuce Wraps

Tandoori Jackfruit and Chutney Panini

Jerk Tofu Wraps

Seitan Gyros with Tzatziki Black Bean Meatball

Subs Pizza Pockets

Cheesy Summer Squash Flatbreads

PREP TIME: 10 minutes

COOK TIME: 15 minutes

NUT-FREE, SOY-FREE

SERVES 4

I love serving this for lunch in the summer when so many great vegetables are in season. Summer squash has a sunshine-like hue that brightens any dish and contrasts nicely with the deep greens of the asparagus and spinach. If summer squash isn't in season, swap it for zucchini instead. You can customize this dish with many other great vegetable combos like spinach, mushroom, and tomato, or use a flavored hummus, like roasted red pepper, to add more flavor.

3 small yellow summer squash, thinly sliced

8 to 10 thin asparagus stalks, trimmed

1 tablespoon grapeseed or extra-virgin olive oil

½ teaspoon salt

2 cups baby spinach

2 vegan naan or flatbreads

⅓ cup hummus

1 cup shredded mozzarella-style vegan cheese

½ teaspoon freshly ground black pepper

1. Preheat the oven to 425°F. Line a rimmed baking sheet with parchment paper.

2. In a large bowl, toss the squash and asparagus with the oil and salt. Arrange on the prepared baking sheet in a single layer and bake for 10 to 12 minutes. Remove from the oven, transfer to a bowl, and toss with the spinach.

3. Replace the parchment paper on the baking sheet with a fresh piece

and lay both pieces of naan on it. Spread the hummus evenly over both breads. Top with the squash, asparagus, and spinach and sprinkle with the cheese. Bake for 2 to 3 minutes, or until the cheese is melted. Sprinkle with pepper just before serving.

INGREDIENT TIP: Yellow summer squash and zucchini are picked when semi-ripe or immature, meaning they have a tender and edible skin. Both are very high in fiber, roast or bake up quickly, and are a delicious addition to your summer vegetable rotation.

PER SERVING: Calories: 289; Fat: 14g; Protein: 7g; Carbohydrates: 35g; Fiber: 5g

Seven-Layer Burritos

PREP TIME: 20 minutes

COOK TIME: 5 minutes

NUT-FREE, ONE POT

SERVES 4

I'll eat almost anything wrapped in a tortilla—including breakfast! It's the ultimate grab-and-go meal. This seven-layer burrito is a fantastic, quick way to get a hearty, filling, veggie-packed meal.

If you don't feel like prepping the Tex-Mex crumble ahead of time, swap it for chickpeas or a store-bought veggie beef crumble. You can also dial up the heat with pickled jalapeño slices or add some store-bought vegan cheese shreds or sour cream.

1 tablespoon grapeseed or extra-virgin olive oil

2 cups Tex-Mex-Style Tofu

1 tablespoon chili powder

4 (10-inch) whole-wheat flour tortillas

1 cup vegetarian refried beans

2 cups shredded iceberg lettuce

⅔ cup mild or medium salsa

½ cup canned corn drained

1 large avocado, peeled, pitted, and diced

1 cup canned black beans, drained and rinsed

1. In a medium skillet, heat the oil over medium-high heat. Add the tofu and chili powder and cook, tossing frequently for 3 to 5 minutes, until warmed through and coated. Alternatively, you can do this in the microwave for 1 to 2 minutes.

2. Lay the tortillas on a flat surface and spread 2 tablespoons of refried beans down the middle of each tortilla in a horizontal line. Building

on top of the beans, add ½ cup of tofu, ½ cup of lettuce, 2 to 3 tablespoons of salsa, 2 tablespoons of corn, a quarter of the avocado, and ¼ cup of black beans.

3. Fold in the left and right sides of your burrito until they almost touch, then bring up the bottom of the tortilla and roll, tucking under as you go, until you've got a burrito shape. Serve immediately.

MAKE IT FASTER: For quick wraps, burritos, and even salads, keep a bag of shredded iceberg lettuce on hand. Bagged lettuce is prewashed and saves tons of prep time when you're in a hurry.

PER SERVING: Calories: 491; Fat: 21g; Protein: 21g; Carbohydrates: 60g; Fiber: 18g

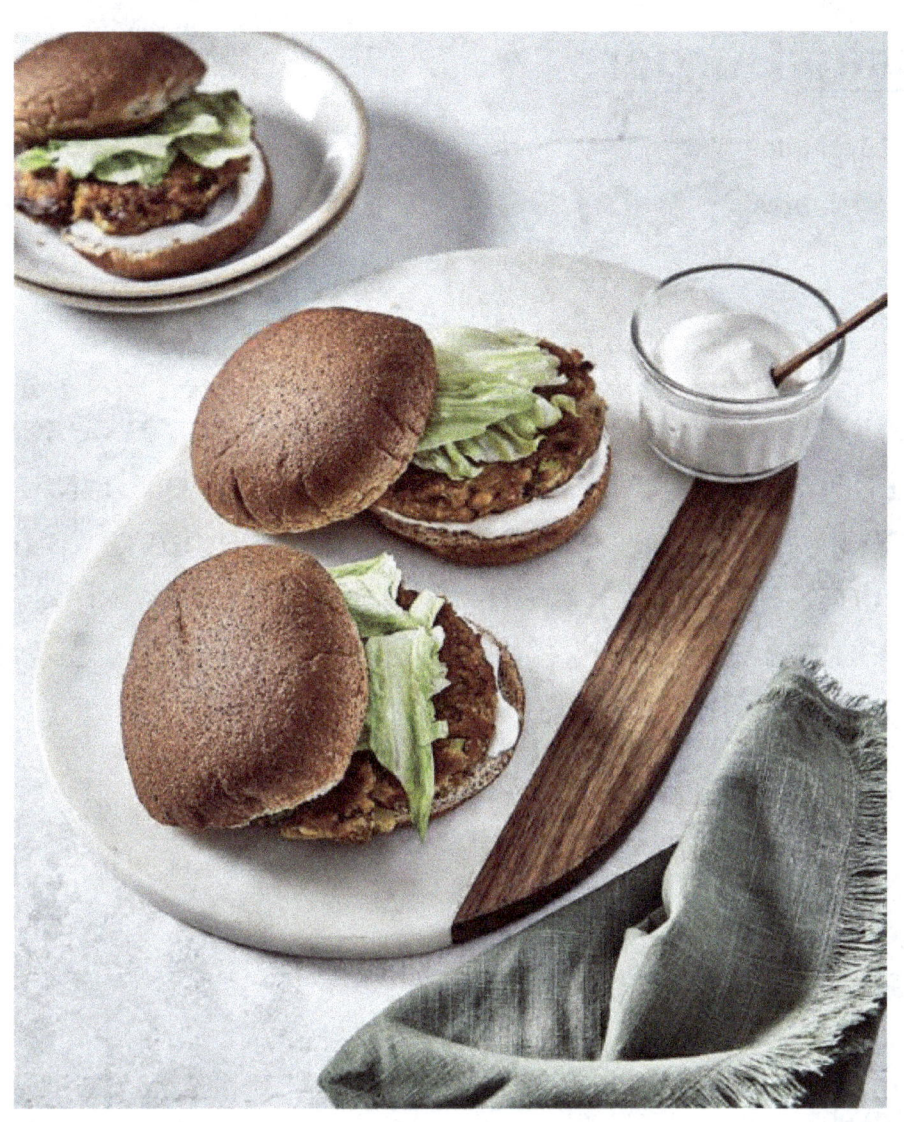

Crab Cake Burgers

PREP TIME: 15 minutes

COOK TIME: 5 minutes

NUT-FREE

SERVES 6

Switch up burger night with these delicious "crab cakes" made from chickpeas and hearts of palm. Because both ingredients are packed in brine, they add a seafood-like flavor to this dish that is reminiscent of real crab. You can use just chickpeas if that's all you have, but I like the addition of hearts of palm, which mimic the shredded texture of crab.

1 (15-ounce) can chickpeas, drained and rinsed

1 (14-ounce) can hearts of palm, drained and coarsely chopped

1 celery stalk, finely diced

2 scallions, both white and green parts, chopped

2 tablespoons Old Bay seasoning

1 tablespoon low-sodium soy sauce

1 teaspoon freshly squeezed lemon juice

¾ cup breadcrumbs

3 tablespoons grapeseed or extra-virgin olive oil

6 whole-wheat or multigrain burger buns

12 large iceberg lettuce leaves

¼ cup Vegan Mayonnaise or store-bought, for topping (optional)

1. In a large bowl, combine the chickpeas and hearts of palm. Using a fork or a potato masher, mash both into small chunks. Alternatively, you could do this in a food processor.

2. Add the celery, scallions, Old Bay, soy sauce, and lemon juice and mix well. Stir in the breadcrumbs. Divide the mixture into 6 even portions and using your hands, form them into patties about ¾ inch thick.

3. In a large sauté pan or skillet, heat the oil on medium-high heat until shimmering. Add the patties and pan-fry for 3 minutes per side, or until crispy on the outside. Serve on burger buns, topped with lettuce and mayonnaise (if using).

PER SERVING: Calories: 325; Fat: 11g; Protein: 13g; Carbohydrates: 46g; Fiber: 8g

Veggie Supreme Garlic Bread Pizza

PREP TIME: 15 minutes

COOK TIME: 10 minutes

NUT-FREE, SOY-FREE

SERVES 4

Ever notice how well pizza and garlic bread go together? Like when you order a pizza online and they always try to upsell you on garlic sticks? Well, what if your pizza was made *on* garlic bread? Take pizza night to a whole new level this weekend with these homemade garlic bread pizzas made on French baguettes with a garlic-butter base and all your favorite toppings.

1 baguette, halved vertically and horizontally to form 4 equal pieces

⅓ cup vegan butter, at room temperature

2 teaspoons minced garlic

1½ cups tomato sauce

½ red bell pepper, finely diced ½

green bell pepper, finely diced

4 large cremini mushrooms, stems removed and caps sliced

⅓ cup sliced black olives

1 cup shredded mozzarella-style vegan cheese

1. Preheat the oven to 400°F. Line a rimmed baking sheet with parchment paper and arrange the baguette pieces in a single layer, cut side up.

2. In a small bowl, stir together the butter and garlic. Spread an even layer of garlic butter on each baguette and bake for 5 to 7 minutes, or until the bread is just lightly golden. Remove from the oven.

3. Spread a thin layer of tomato sauce on top, add the peppers, mushrooms, and olives, and then sprinkle with the cheese. Bake for

another 3 to 5 minutes, or until the cheese is melted, then serve.

PER SERVING: Calories: 382; Fat: 23g; Protein: 6g; Carbohydrates: 40g; Fiber: 2g

Cashew Curry Tofu Pita Pockets

PREP TIME: 15 minutes

NO COOK, SUPERFAST

SERVES 4

This salad is a riff on a curry chicken salad I grew up eating from a favorite childhood deli. I've made it several different ways, by roasting and dicing store-bought vegan chick'n strips, using baked tofu, and even chickpeas, which is a great alternative if you're avoiding soy. The combination of heat from the curry powder, tartness from the apples, cranberries, and lime juice, and crunch from the cashews gives this sandwich great texture and flavor.

1 (14-ounce) block extra-firm tofu, drained, pressed, and grated on the large side of a box grater

1 tart apple (such as Granny Smith), cored and diced

¾ cup roasted unsalted cashews

2 celery stalks, finely diced

½ cup dried cranberries

3 to 4 tablespoons Vegan Mayonnaise or store-bought 2 tablespoons mild curry powder

Juice of ½ lime

½ teaspoon freshly ground black pepper

4 whole-wheat pocket-style pitas, halved

8 large iceberg or Bibb lettuce leaves

1. In a large bowl, combine the tofu, apple, cashews, celery, cranberries, mayonnaise, curry powder, lime juice, and pepper and mix to combine. Taste and adjust the seasoning if necessary.

2. Line each pita pocket with one large lettuce leaf and add a large scoop of the cashew curry tofu mix. Serve.

PER SERVING: Calories: 554; Fat: 24g; Protein: 21g; Carbohydrates: 70g; Fiber: 10g

Tofu-Lettuce-Tomato-Avocado Sandwich

PREP TIME: 15 minutes

COOK TIME: 15 minutes

NUT-FREE

SERVES 4

I promise that once you try this smoked tofu "bacon," it will become your new go-to dish. It's the perfect side to your morning tofu scramble or pancakes, a salad topping on the Caesar Pasta Salad, or a component in this vegan BLT. The addition of liquid smoke to the marinade adds an authentic smoked bacon flavor, but it's not absolutely necessary, as the tofu will still be delicious without it.

2 tablespoons low-sodium soy sauce

1 tablespoon maple syrup

1 teaspoon apple cider vinegar

3 drops liquid smoke (optional)

1 tablespoon grapeseed or extra-virgin olive oil

1 (14-ounce) block extra-firm tofu, drained, pressed, and cut into ½-inch-thick slices

8 slices multigrain or whole-wheat bread, toasted

4 tablespoons Vegan Mayonnaise or store-bought

8 large iceberg lettuce leaves

1 large hothouse tomato, sliced

1 large avocado, peeled, pitted, and sliced

1. In a small bowl, combine the soy sauce, maple syrup, vinegar, and liquid smoke (if using). Set aside.

2. In a large sauté pan or skillet, heat the oil over medium-high heat. Once the oil is hot, add the tofu slices and pan-fry for 7 to 10 minutes, or until the tofu is golden brown on both sides. Add the marinade to the pan and cook for 2 to 3 minutes, or until almost all the liquid is gone and the tofu is sticky and caramelized.

3. Spread ½ tablespoon of mayonnaise on each slice of toast. Add 2 lettuce leaves and a quarter of the smoked tofu to 4 of the toasts. Layer on the tomato and avocado slices. Top each sandwich with another piece of toast and serve.

PER SERVING: Calories: 547; Fat: 27g; Protein: 23g; Carbohydrates: 58g; Fiber: 16g

Spinach and Mushroom Baguettes with Garlic-Herb Cream Cheese

PREP TIME: 5 minutes

COOK TIME: 10 minutes

EASY PREP, NUT-FREE, SUPERFAST

SERVES 4

When I need dinner in a hurry, or a show-stopping appetizer in no time at all, I make this dish, and it's always a crowd pleaser. The earthiness of mushrooms and spinach with soy sauce perfectly complements the richness of the cream cheese. For a dinner serving, I like to use bigger Italian bread slices, but if I'm serving this as an appetizer, a French baguette makes the perfect two-bite snack.

2 tablespoons grapeseed or extra-virgin olive oil

2 cups sliced white button or cremini mushrooms

2 pounds fresh spinach

1 teaspoon minced garlic

1 teaspoon low-sodium soy sauce

½ cup Garlic and Herb Tofu Cream Cheese or store-bought

1 French or Italian demi-baguette, cut into 8 slices (1½ inches wide),
toasted Sea salt

Freshly ground black pepper

1. In a large sauté pan or skillet, heat the oil on medium-high heat. Add the mushrooms and cook for about 5 minutes, until they start to get dark and golden. Add the spinach, garlic, and soy sauce and continue to cook, stirring frequently, until the spinach is wilted and the mushrooms are softened, another 3 to 5 minutes.

2. Spread about 2 tablespoons of cream cheese on each toasted baguette and top with the vegetable mixture. Season with salt and pepper to taste and serve.

SMART SHOPPING: Choose prewashed bagged spinach and a jar of minced garlic, and you can get this dish on the table in just a few minutes.

PER SERVING: Calories: 259; Fat: 11g; Protein: 14g; Carbohydrates: 31g; Fiber: 7g

Tofu Fish Tacos

PREP TIME: 20 minutes

COOK TIME: 10 minutes

NUT-FREE

SERVES 2

Give Taco Tuesday new life with these tofu "fish" tacos. I like to cut the tofu into triangles, but you could also dice the tofu into 1-inch cubes (which stretches this recipe from 2 servings to 4).

4 tablespoons Vegan Mayonnaise or store-bought

2 tablespoons sriracha or other hot sauce

Juice of ½ lime

1 teaspoon ground cumin

1 teaspoon paprika

½ teaspoon kelp flakes

¼ teaspoon salt

¼ teaspoon freshly ground black pepper ⅛ to ¼ teaspoon ground cayenne pepper

1 (14-ounce) block firm tofu, drained and pressed 3 tablespoons grapeseed or extra-virgin olive oil ¼ cup plus 2 tablespoons cornstarch

4 medium whole-wheat flour tortillas

1 cup shredded iceberg lettuce or lettuce/ cabbage mix

1. In a small bowl, combine the mayonnaise and sriracha, stirring well to make a spicy mayonnaise sauce. Set aside.
2. In a large dish, combine the lime juice, cumin, paprika, kelp, salt, black pepper, and cayenne. Mix well.
3. Cut the tofu in half, then slice each piece in half lengthwise so that you have 4 equal square pieces. Cut each square in half diagonally to create a total of 8 triangles. Place the tofu in the dish with the

marinade and turn to coat. Refrigerate for 10 minutes.

4. In a large sauté pan or skillet, heat the oil on medium-high heat, swirling to coat the pan. When hot, reduce the heat to medium. Place the cornstarch in a shallow bowl, and remove tofu from the refrigerator. Dip each piece of tofu in the cornstarch, then place in the hot pan. Cook for 5 minutes per side, or until crispy and lightly browned.

5. Add two tofu triangles to each tortilla, top with lettuce, and drizzle with the spicy mayonnaise.

INGREDIENT TIP: Kelp flakes add a briny flavor to dishes in place of fish or seafood. You can find them (or dulce flakes—a close cousin of kelp) in the seafood sections of many mainstream grocery stores.

PER SERVING: Calories: 871; Fat: 51g; Protein: 28g; Carbohydrates: 79g; Fiber: 9g

Kung Pao Tempeh Lettuce Wraps

PREP TIME: 10 minutes

COOK TIME: 10 minutes

GLUTEN-FREE, NUT-FREE

SERVES 3

I adore lettuce wraps. The fresh, cool crunch of lettuce is a welcome change from carb-based wrappers, especially on hot summer days. The filling for these wraps is easy to make and packs a lot of punch. Adding water chestnuts to this dish adds great texture and crunch. You'll typically find them in the international aisle of your grocery store, but if you can't, swap them out for a couple of stalks of diced celery instead.

1 tablespoon grapeseed or extra-virgin olive oil

1 (7-ounce) package tempeh, crumbled

1 red bell pepper, diced

1 (8-ounce) can sliced water chestnuts, drained and diced ¼ cup low-sodium vegetable broth

3 scallions, both white and green parts, chopped

1 tablespoon tamari

2 teaspoons maple syrup

1 teaspoon chili paste, such as sriracha or sambal oelek

1 teaspoon white vinegar

2 tablespoons cold water

1 tablespoon cornstarch

8 to 10 whole iceberg lettuce cups

1. In a large sauté pan or skillet, heat the oil on medium-high heat. Add the tempeh and bell pepper and cook for 3 to 5 minutes, or until the tempeh is warmed through.

2. Add the water chestnuts, vegetable broth, scallions, tamari, maple syrup, chili paste, and vinegar and stir to combine.

3. In a small dish, whisk together the water and cornstarch. Add it to the tempeh mixture and stir to combine. Simmer until the sauce is thickened and absorbed by the tempeh, about 5 minutes. Spoon into lettuce cups to serve.

PER SERVING: Calories: 231; Fat: 12g; Protein: 16g; Carbohydrates: 20g; Fiber: 5g

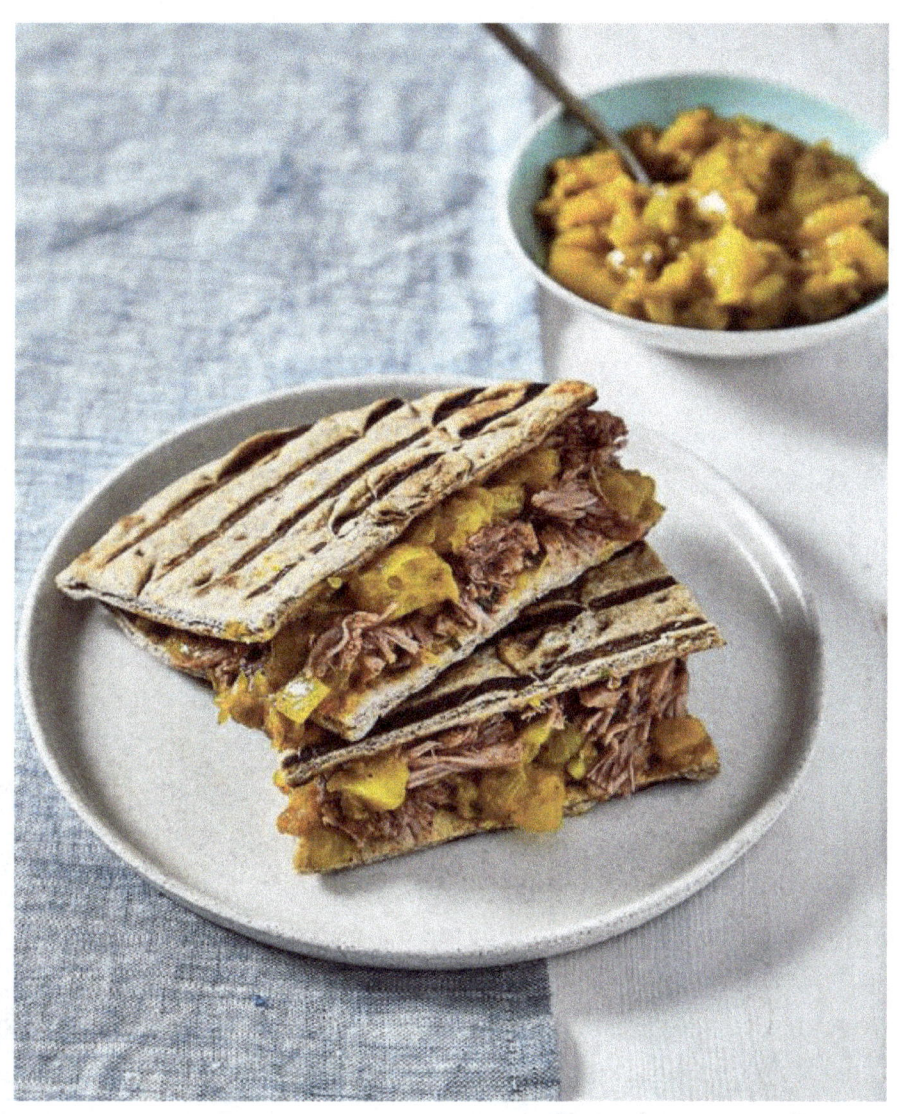

Tandoori Jackfruit and Chutney Panini

PREP TIME: 10 minutes

COOK TIME: 15 minutes

SOY-FREE

SERVES 4

I love the contrast of spicy and sweet in this sandwich. The tandoori seasoning is wicked hot and is tempered by the yogurt and the sweetness of mango chutney. Jackfruit is a tree fruit from India and Malaysia that is often used in vegan cooking for its meaty texture. Shred the jackfruit using your hands or pull it apart with two forks. It will also naturally break down and shred easily in the pan as it cooks.

1 tablespoon grapeseed or extra-virgin olive oil

3 scallions, both green and white parts, chopped and divided

1 (14-ounce) can young jackfruit packed in brine or water, drained and shredded ½ cup low-sodium vegetable broth

2 tablespoons tandoori masala paste, such as Rani

2 tablespoons unsweetened coconut yogurt

4 tablespoons Mango Chutney or store-bought

4 vegan naan or pita, halved

1. In a large sauté pan or skillet, heat the oil on medium-high heat. Add half of the scallions and cook for 1 to 2 minutes, or until fragrant. Add the jackfruit, vegetable broth, and tandoori paste. Simmer on medium heat until the jackfruit is soft and most of the liquid is absorbed, about 10 minutes.

2. Remove from the heat and stir in the yogurt and remaining scallions.

3. Spread 1 tablespoon of chutney on each piece of naan. Top with about ¼ cup of jackfruit and cover with the remaining pieces of naan. Grill in a panini press or in a pan on the stove on medium-high heat

for 3 to 4 minutes per side.

INGREDIENT TIP: If you can't find tandoori paste, you can use a dry tandoori spice mix instead. In a small bowl, combine 3 tablespoons of paprika, 1 tablespoon of turmeric, and 1 teaspoon each of garlic powder, ground nutmeg, cayenne pepper, ground ginger, ground coriander, ground cumin, and ground cloves. Use 1 tablespoon for this recipe and store the rest in an airtight container in your pantry for up to 4 months. Recipe yields ⅓ cup of spice mix.

PER SERVING: Calories: 309; Fat: 9g; Protein: 8g; Carbohydrates: 49g; Fiber: 10g

Jerk Tofu Wraps

PREP TIME: 10 minutes

COOK TIME: 20 minutes

NUT-FREE

SERVES 3

Don't let the ingredient list in this recipe scare you—it's really easy to make. I've included a recipe for homemade jerk seasoning (hence the long ingredient list), but you could always use a store-bought jerk spice rub or marinade here instead. If you are making the homemade version below, I highly recommend doubling the recipe and storing half of it, as it's fabulous on roasted cauliflower or as a twist on my Basic Seitan.

For the jerk seasoning

1 to 2 tablespoons ground cayenne pepper

1 tablespoon onion powder

1 tablespoon garlic powder

1 tablespoon brown sugar

1 tablespoon dried parsley

2 teaspoons smoked or regular paprika

1 teaspoon freshly ground black pepper

1 teaspoon ground cinnamon

1 teaspoon ground nutmeg

1 teaspoon dried thyme

½ teaspoon red pepper flakes

½ teaspoon ground cumin

For the tofu wraps

1 (14-ounce) block extra-firm tofu, drained, pressed, and cut into 1-inch cubes

1 tablespoon cornstarch

2 tablespoons grapeseed or extra-virgin olive oil

½ medium onion, sliced

½ red bell pepper, sliced

½ green bell pepper, sliced

1 cup pineapple chunks, fresh or canned

4 large (10-inch) whole-wheat tortillas

2 cups spring mix salad greens

1. To make the jerk seasoning: In a large resealable bag, combine the cayenne, onion powder, garlic powder, brown sugar, parsley, paprika, black pepper, cinnamon, nutmeg, thyme, red pepper flakes, and cumin.

2. Add the tofu and cornstarch, seal the bag, and shake until the tofu is well coated.

3. In a large sauté pan or skillet, heat the oil on medium-high heat. Add the onion and peppers and cook for 5 minutes, or until the onion is slightly translucent and the peppers begin to soften.

4. Scoop the tofu out of the bag and add it to the pan. Cook for 10 to 15 minutes, or until the tofu is crispy. Remove the pan from the heat and stir in the pineapple chunks.

5. Divide the salad leaves evenly among the tortillas and top each with one-quarter of the jerk tofu. Fold in the sides of the tortillas, then roll up, starting from the bottom. Slice in half and serve.

INGREDIENT TIP: Jerk is a style of cooking that is native to Jamaica and involves using a dry rub or a wet marinade to season and coat a protein (usually meat) before cooking, usually over a grill. What sets jerk seasoning apart from other spicy rubs or marinades is the use of allspice and Scotch bonnet peppers, both of which can easily be added to the homemade jerk seasoning in this recipe.

PER SERVING: Calories: 553; Fat: 23g; Protein: 24g; Carbohydrates: 72g; Fiber: 14g

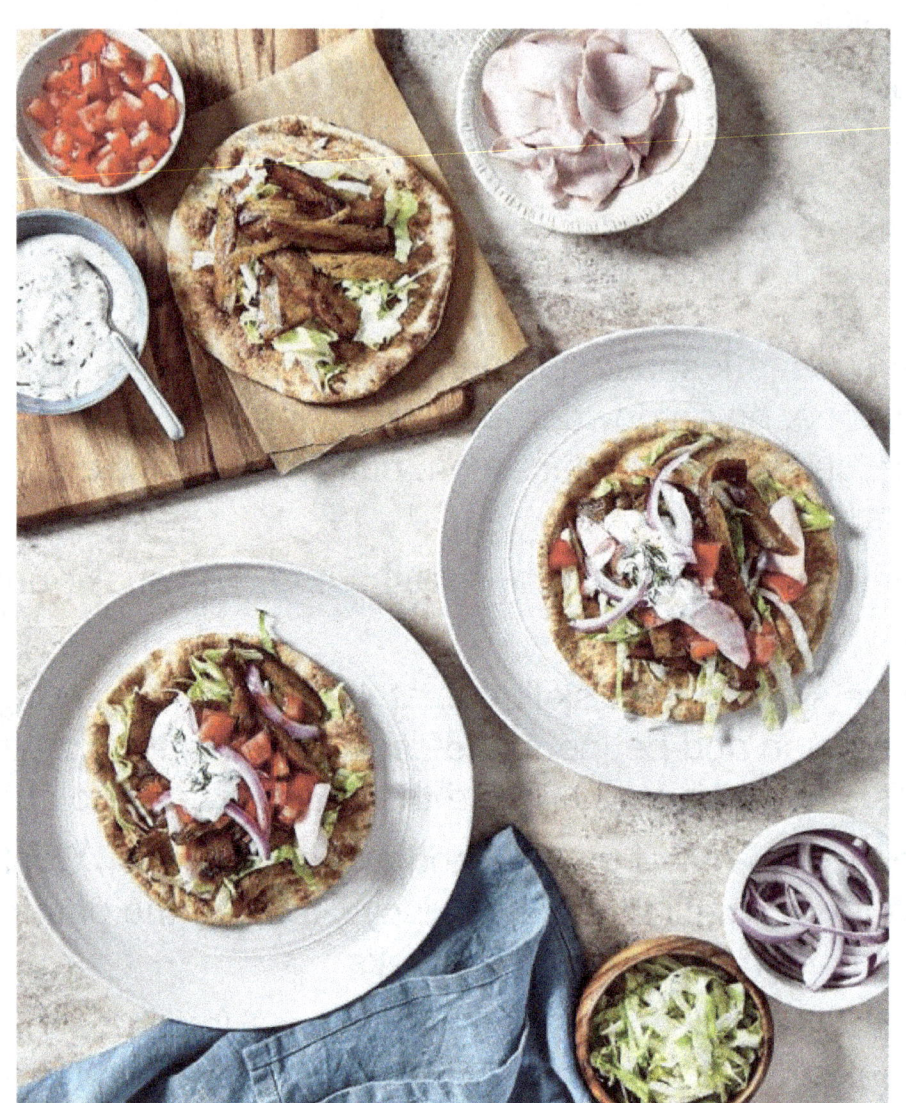

Seitan Gyros with Tzatziki

PREP TIME: 10 minutes

COOK TIME: 20 minutes

NUT-FREE

SERVES 6

This dish is a play on the traditional vertical rotisserie dish popular in Greek cooking. Seitan, a vegan meat substitute made from wheat gluten, mimics the traditional gyro meat. Top it with a vegan tzatziki that has fooled even the most hardcore non-vegans.

¼ seedless cucumber ⅔
cup vegan sour cream

⅓ cup Vegan Mayonnaise or store-
bought 1 tablespoon chopped fresh dill

1 tablespoon freshly squeezed lemon juice

1 teaspoon grated lemon zest

1 teaspoon freshly ground black pepper

1 teaspoon salt

½ teaspoon minced garlic

½ teaspoon onion powder

2 tablespoons grapeseed or extra-virgin olive oil

1 recipe Basic Seitan, sliced thin or shaved

1½ cups shredded iceberg lettuce

6 (10-inch) whole-wheat tortillas or
pitas 2 plum tomatoes, diced

¼ red onion, sliced

½ cup pickled turnips

Hot sauce (optional)

1. Using a box grater with large holes, grate the cucumber and squeeze it to release as much water as possible, then place in a medium bowl. Add the sour cream, mayonnaise, dill, lemon juice and zest, pepper,

salt, garlic, and onion powder. Whisk or stir well to combine. Refrigerate while you fry the seitan.

2. In a large sauté pan or skillet, heat the oil on medium-high heat. Once hot, add the seitan slices a few at a time, being careful not to crowd the pan. Cook for 3 minutes per side, until lightly browned. Repeat until all the seitan is cooked.

3. Divide the lettuce evenly between the tortillas. Add 6 to 8 slices of seitan, then top with the tomatoes, onion, turnips, and a tablespoon of tzatziki. Add a dash or two of hot sauce (if using). Roll up and serve.

DIETARY TIP: Make this dish gluten-free by swapping out the seitan gyros for roasted vegetables like cauliflower, zucchini, and peppers, and use a gluten-free wrap. Use some olive oil and the spices from the Basic Seitan to give your veggies that authentic gyro taste.

PER SERVING: Calories: 499; Fat: 21g; Protein: 36g; Carbohydrates: 53g; Fiber: 13g

Black Bean Meatball Subs

PREP TIME: 15 minutes

COOK TIME: 15 minutes

NUT-FREE, SOY-FREE

SERVES 4

In the same amount of time as it would take to head to your favorite sub shop and order dinner, you can have these authentic, homemade meatless Italian meatball subs on the table. Made from black beans and mushrooms for a meaty, earthy taste, these meatballs are also delicious served with spaghetti and a side salad.

1 (15-ounce) can black beans, drained, ¼ cup liquid reserved

1 cup panko breadcrumbs

3 or 4 cremini mushrooms, coarsely chopped

4 teaspoons Italian seasoning

1 teaspoon minced garlic

1 teaspoon onion powder

1 teaspoon cornstarch

½ teaspoon salt

½ teaspoon freshly ground black

pepper ¼ teaspoon red pepper flakes

2 tablespoons grapeseed or extra-virgin olive oil

1 (24-ounce) jar marinara sauce

4 Italian sub rolls or sausage buns, sliced open

1 cup shredded mozzarella-style vegan cheese

1. In a food processor fitted with the steel blade, combine the beans, reserved bean liquid, breadcrumbs, mushrooms, Italian seasoning, garlic, onion powder, cornstarch, salt, black pepper, and red pepper flakes. Process until a smooth, sticky mixture forms. Remove the blade and set aside.

2. In a large sauté pan or skillet, heat the oil on medium-high heat. Scoop out the black bean mixture in scant ¼-cup amounts and roll into balls. Place in the hot skillet and cook until the bottoms are brown, about 5 minutes, then flip and cook the other side for another 5 minutes.

3. When all the meatballs are cooked, add the marinara sauce to the pan and simmer the sauce and meatballs for 5 minutes, or until the sauce is warm.

4. Place 3 meatballs in each roll, drizzle with sauce, and top with the cheese.

VARY IT: You can switch up the seasonings and work these meatballs into your meal plans in a number of ways. Replace the Italian seasoning with chili powder, ground cumin, and paprika for a great Tex-Mex flavor. Or opt for cumin, smoked paprika, coriander, and sumac for a Middle Eastern flair.

PER SERVING: Calories: 623; Fat: 18g; Protein: 19g; Carbohydrates: 101g; Fiber: 14g

Pizza Pockets

PREP TIME: 10 minutes

COOK TIME: 20 minutes

NUT-FREE, SOY-FREE

SERVES 4

Pizza pockets were an integral part of my childhood. They were the best. And while frozen vegan versions probably do exist, they aren't nearly as healthy, good, or inexpensive as homemade. I use store-bought pizza dough to turn this childhood favorite into a quick and easy grown-up meal that bakes in the time it takes to make a quick salad. Try adding my Meat-Free Pepperoni or your favorite vegan sausage to make this a supreme pocket.

All-purpose flour, for rolling

1 (1-pound) ball store-bought pizza dough

1 cup marinara sauce

½ cup shredded mozzarella-style vegan cheese

½ cup sliced mushrooms

½ cup sliced green bell pepper

½ cup sliced red onion

2 tablespoons grapeseed or extra-virgin olive oil

1 tablespoon Italian seasoning

1. Preheat the oven to 425°F. Line a rimmed baking sheet with parchment paper and set aside.

2. On a floured surface, roll out the dough into a rectangle about ½ inch thick. Cut into 8 rectangles. On one half of each rectangle, add about 1 tablespoon of marinara sauce and top with 1 tablespoon each of cheese, mushrooms, green peppers, and onion. Fold, sealing all edges by pressing them down with a fork, and transfer to the prepared baking sheet.

3. In a small bowl, mix together the oil and Italian seasoning. Gently brush the tops of each pizza pocket with the seasoned oil.

4. Bake for 20 minutes, until the dough looks crisp and golden. Serve immediately.

PER SERVING: Calories: 415; Fat: 14g; Protein: 8g; Carbohydrates: 62g; Fiber: 4g

5

Pasta and Noodles

Tofu Pad Thai
Creamy Garlic Penne
Tex-Mex Mac and Cheese
Pizza-Night Penne
Pad See Ew
Spinach and Ricotta Stuffed Shells Fiery
Linguini with Spinach and Peas Curry
Penne with Mango Chutney Burst Cherry
Tomato Rigatoni Pasta Primavera
Creamy Sun-Dried Tomato and Spinach Pasta
Vegetable Lo Mein
Singapore-Style Vermicelli
Udon Noodles with Mushrooms and Cabbage
Creamy Cajun Mushroom Pasta

Tofu Pad Thai

PREP TIME: 15 minutes

COOK TIME: 15 minutes

GLUTEN-FREE

SERVES 4

This dish is a family favorite of ours and my saving grace on busy weeknights when I haven't meal-planned or am short on time. The sauce comes together while the noodles cook, and the tofu and vegetables only take a few minutes in the pan on high heat, so no matter how rushed you are, you can have a great dinner in under 30 minutes.

1 (13-ounce) package pad Thai rice noodles

½ cup sweet Thai chili

sauce ¼ cup tamari

2 tablespoons creamy peanut butter

1 tablespoon sugar

2 teaspoons minced

garlic Juice of 1 lime

½ cup full-fat coconut milk

1 tablespoon grapeseed or extra-virgin olive oil

1 (14-ounce) block extra-firm tofu, drained, pressed, and cut into 1-inch cubes

½ medium onion, cut into strips

½ red bell pepper, cut into strips

1 cup (packed) bean sprouts

1. Bring a large pot of water to a boil and cook the noodles according to package directions.

2. While the noodles are cooking, in a small bowl, combine the chili sauce, tamari, peanut butter, sugar, garlic, and lime juice. Whisk until smooth. Add the coconut milk and stir to incorporate.

3. Drain and rinse the noodles under cold water to keep them from

sticking. Set aside.

4. In a large sauté pan or skillet, heat the oil on medium-high heat. Add the tofu, onion, and bell pepper and stir-fry for 7 to 8 minutes, until the tofu is golden and the onion and bell pepper are soft.

5. Add the rice noodles, sauce, and bean sprouts and toss to combine. Cook for 1 to 2 minutes, or until the noodles are warmed through, and serve.

VARY IT: Turn this sauce into a fabulous dip for spring rolls, fresh rice paper rolls, or tofu satay. Make the sauce per the instructions above, leaving out the coconut milk.

PER SERVING: Calories: 690; Fat: 18g; Protein: 21g; Carbohydrates: 102g; Fiber: 5g

Creamy Garlic Penne

PREP TIME: 5 minutes

COOK TIME: 10 minutes

EASY PREP, NUT-FREE, SUPERFAST

SERVES 6

I love this recipe for its simplicity. The rich, creamy garlic sauce tastes like it simmered for hours, but comes together in the time it takes the penne to cook, meaning you spend less time cooking and more time enjoying. My youngest daughter loves broccoli so I like to drop 1 to 2 cups of broccoli florets into the cooking pasta for the last two minutes of cook time.

1 (16-ounce) box penne pasta

4 tablespoons vegan butter

6 garlic cloves, minced

¼ cup all-purpose flour

1½ cups low-sodium vegetable broth

1½ cups unsweetened soy milk

½ cup nutritional yeast or vegan Parmesan cheese 1 tablespoon dried parsley

¼ teaspoon salt

¼ teaspoon freshly ground black pepper

1. Bring a large pot of water to a boil and cook the pasta according to package directions.

2. While the pasta is cooking, in a large sauté pan or skillet, melt the butter over medium heat. Add the garlic and cook, stirring constantly, for 1 to 2 minutes, until the garlic is fragrant but not dark. Add the flour and cook for 1 to 2 minutes, stirring constantly, until the flour has been absorbed into the butter, forming a roux.

3. Slowly add the vegetable broth and soy milk to the pan, stirring constantly, until the sauce begins to boil and thicken, about 5

minutes. Stir in the nutritional yeast, parsley, salt, and pepper.

4. Drain the pasta and add it to the pan. Toss to coat.

PER SERVING: Calories: 436; Fat: 10g; Protein: 18g; Carbohydrates: 67g; Fiber: 6g

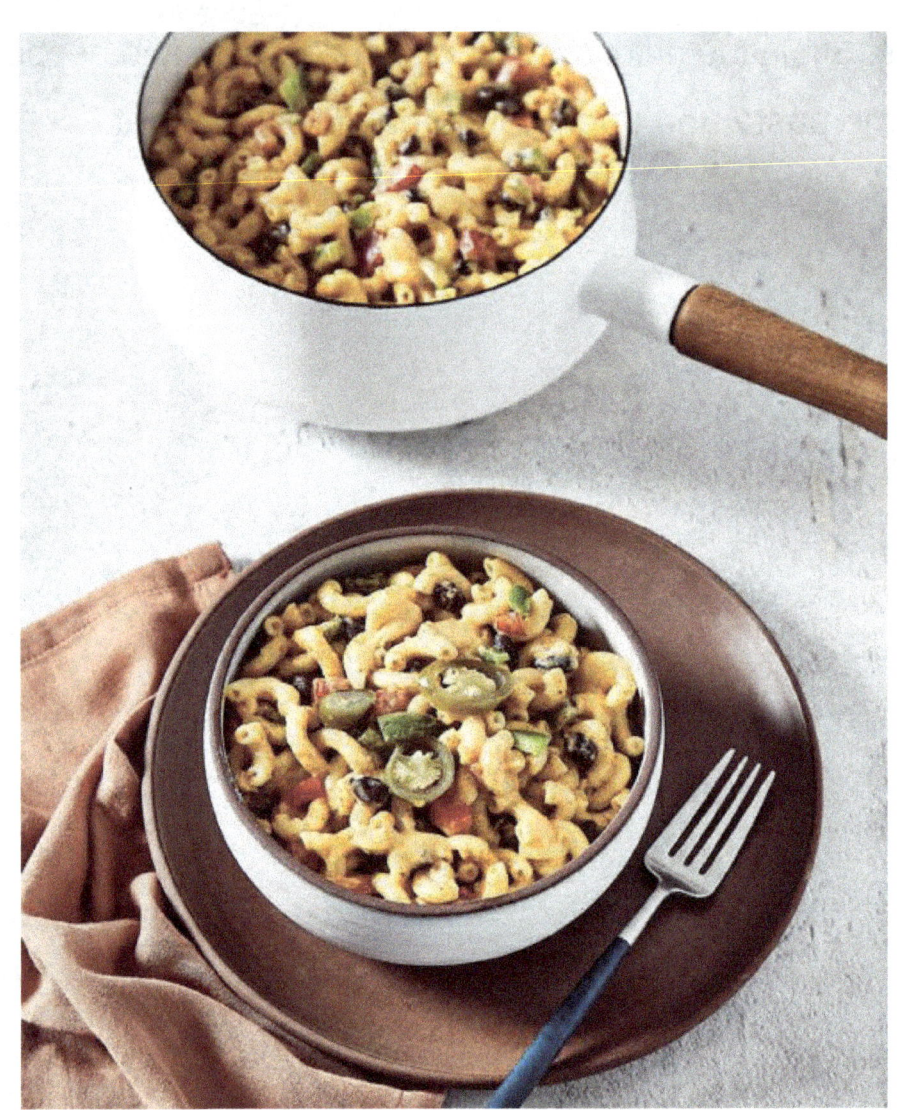

Tex-Mex Mac and Cheese

PREP TIME: 5 minutes

COOK TIME: 10 minutes

EASY PREP, NUT-FREE, ONE POT, SUPERFAST

SERVES 4

This is a fun twist on a classic stovetop mac and cheese. All the prep can be done while the pasta is cooking, which keeps this dish easy for weeknight meals. I like to serve this with a salad and a creamy vegan ranch dressing. If you have any flavored vegan cream cheese, like onion, chive, or garlic, add a tablespoon to this dish to make the sauce even more flavorful and creamy.

1 (16-ounce) box elbow macaroni
1 cup unsweetened soy milk
½ cup Cheddar-Style Cheese Sauce or shredded Cheddar-style vegan cheese 2 tablespoons vegan butter
2 tablespoons nutritional yeast
1 tablespoon chili powder or taco seasoning
1 cup canned black beans, drained and rinsed
½ red bell pepper, diced
½ green bell pepper, diced
Sliced pickled jalapeño peppers, for garnish (optional)

1. Bring a large pot of water to a boil and cook the pasta according to pasta directions. Drain and return to the pot.

2. Add the soy milk, cheese sauce, butter, nutritional yeast, and chili powder to the cooked pasta and stir to combine until the milk is absorbed and the pasta is coated. Add the black beans and bell peppers and stir to combine. Top with jalapeño peppers (if using) and serve.

VARY IT: Add some [Tex-Mex-Style Tofu](#) to make this dish into a true chili mac and cheese.

PER SERVING: Calories: 617; Fat: 11g; Protein: 24g; Carbohydrates: 105g; Fiber: 12g

Pizza-Night Penne

PREP TIME: 10 minutes

COOK TIME: 20 minutes

NUT-FREE

SERVES 4

Switch up pizza night into pizza-pasta night! This dish combines all the flavors of your favorite veggie supreme pizza in a rich, creamy pasta dish that is sure to become a family favorite. You can serve this pasta directly from the pot, but I like to top it with extra vegan cheese and bake it for 5 minutes at a high temperature to get a nice, cheesy, bubbly crust on top.

1 (16-ounce) box penne pasta

1 tablespoon grapeseed or extra-virgin olive oil

8 cremini mushrooms, stems removed and caps sliced

1 green bell pepper, sliced

½ red onion, sliced

1 cup unsweetened soy milk

1 cup Cheddar-Style Cheese Sauce or shredded Cheddar-style vegan cheese, divided

2 tablespoons vegan butter

2 tablespoons nutritional yeast

1 tablespoon Italian seasoning

1 cup marinara sauce

1. Preheat the oven to 425°F.

2. Bring a large pot of water to a boil and cook the pasta according to package directions. Drain and return to the pot.

3. While the pasta is cooking, in a medium-size pan, heat the oil and cook the mushrooms, bell pepper, and onion until soft, about 5 minutes. Remove from the heat.

4. To the cooked pasta, add the soy milk, ½ cup of cheese sauce, butter,

nutritional yeast, and Italian seasoning. Stir until the pasta is coated.

5. Add the cooked vegetables and marinara sauce. Transfer to an oven-safe 9-by-13-inch baking dish, top with the remaining ½ cup of cheese sauce, and bake for 5 minutes, or until the cheese is melted, then serve.

VARY IT: Are you a pepperoni pizza fan? Add some Meat-Free Pepperoni to this pasta dish. I like to add some slices to the prepared pasta in the pot and then top the dish with a layer of pepperoni just before baking.

PER SERVING: Calories: 672; Fat: 18g; Protein: 24g; Carbohydrates: 105g; Fiber: 9g

Pad See Ew

PREP TIME: 10 minutes

COOK TIME: 10 minutes

SERVES 4

Pad see ew, or stir-fried rice noodles with soy sauce, is a classic Thai dish. Most restaurants use fish or oyster sauce in this dish, so I created this plant-based version instead. Traditionally, pad see ew is made with Chinese broccoli (also called gai lan), but if you can't find it, use bok choy, broccolini, or broccoli steamed florets.

1 (16-ounce) package wide rice noodles

3 tablespoons hoisin sauce

2 tablespoons low-sodium soy sauce

1 tablespoon light brown sugar, maple syrup, or agave nectar

1 teaspoon red pepper flakes

1 tablespoon grapeseed or extra-virgin olive oil

2 scallions, both white and green parts, chopped and divided

1 tablespoon water

1 teaspoon minced garlic

12 ounces Chinese broccoli, cut into 2-inch pieces

¼ cup crushed peanuts, for garnish

(optional) Lime wedges, for garnish

Sriracha or other hot sauce, for garnish (optional)

1. Bring a large pot of water to a boil and cook the rice noodles according to package directions. Drain and rinse under cold water to keep them from sticking.

2. While the noodles are cooking, in a small bowl, whisk the hoisin sauce, soy sauce, brown sugar, and red pepper flakes to combine.

3. In a large sauté pan or skillet, heat the oil on medium-high heat. Add the white parts of the scallions and cook for 2 minutes, or until

fragrant. Add the water and garlic and cook for 30 seconds, stirring occasionally.

4. Add the Chinese broccoli and cook for about 3 minutes, until tender and crispy. Add the rice noodles and sauce to the pan and toss to coat. Cook until the noodles are warmed through, about 2 minutes.

5. Top with the green scallions and peanuts (if using) and serve with lime wedges and hot sauce (if using).

VARY IT: Boost your veggie intake by adding fresh green peas, snow peas, or edamame, to this dish.

PER SERVING: Calories: 508; Fat: 5g; Protein: 9g; Carbohydrates: 103g; Fiber: 5g

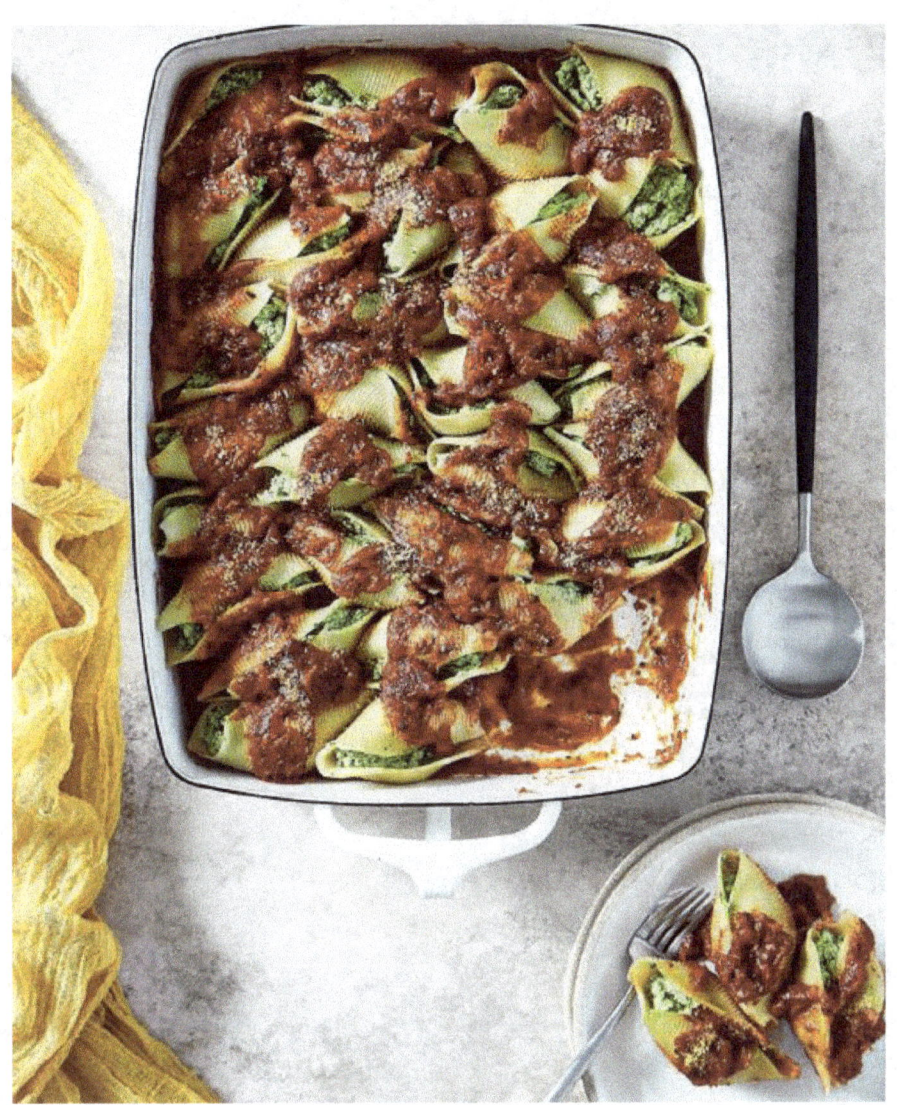

Spinach and Ricotta Stuffed Shells

PREP TIME: 10 minutes

COOK TIME: 15 minutes

NUT-FREE

SERVES 4

Shake up pasta night with jumbo pasta shells, stuffed with a homemade tangy vegan ricotta, drizzled with marinara sauce, and topped with nutritional yeast (or store-bought vegan Parmesan). This vegan ricotta is also great in lasagna. The recipe below will make enough for one layer of ricotta in a standard lasagna.

1 (12-ounce) box jumbo pasta shells

1 (16-ounce) bag baby spinach

1 (14-ounce) block firm or extra-firm tofu, drained, pressed, and cut into 8 pieces

2 tablespoons freshly squeezed lemon juice

1 tablespoon apple cider vinegar

1 teaspoon low-sodium soy sauce

½ teaspoon salt

½ teaspoon freshly ground black pepper

1 (24-ounce) jar marinara sauce

3 tablespoons nutritional yeast

1. Preheat the oven to 400°F.

2. Bring a large pot of water to a boil and cook the pasta according to package directions. When finished, drain and rinse under cold water for 1 minute.

3. While the pasta is cooking, in a food processor fitted with the steel blade, combine the spinach, tofu, lemon juice, apple cider vinegar, soy sauce, salt, and pepper. Process until creamy. Transfer the mixture to a bowl.

4. Scoop a tablespoon of the filling into each shell and place the shells in a 9-by-13-inch baking dish. Drizzle some marinara sauce over each shell and pour the remaining sauce in the dish around the shells. Sprinkle the tops with nutritional yeast.

5. Bake for 5 to 7 minutes, or until the sauce is bubbling. Serve immediately.

VARY IT: If you don't mind adding a few extra minutes to your prep and cook time, pan-fry ½ medium onion, chopped, and 1 cup sliced cremini mushrooms in 1 tablespoon of oil for 5 to 7 minutes, or until the mushrooms are dark. Add them to the food processor with the other ricotta ingredients and blend.

PER SERVING: Calories: 577; Fat: 11g; Protein: 30g; Carbohydrates: 92g; Fiber: 11g

Fiery Linguini with Spinach and Peas

PREP TIME: 5 minutes

COOK TIME: 15 minutes

EASY PREP, SOY-FREE

SERVES 8

My fiery linguini is a play on the classic penne arrabbiata, which translates to "angry pasta." It gets its name from the amount of red pepper flakes in the sauce. This version uses a long noodle instead of the classic tube-shaped pasta; its heat and flavor is just as strong. The sauce is a beautiful orange-red that contrasts nicely against the dark green spinach and bright peas, which add color and nutrients to this dish.

1 (16-ounce) box whole-wheat linguini

1 tablespoon grapeseed or extra-virgin olive oil

1 tablespoon nutritional yeast, plus extra for garnish

1 teaspoon red pepper flakes

1 teaspoon garlic powder

1 teaspoon onion powder

½ teaspoon salt

½ teaspoon freshly ground black

pepper 5 tablespoons tomato paste

3 tablespoons low-sodium vegetable broth

1 (13.5-ounce) can full-fat coconut milk

1 (16-ounce) bag prewashed baby spinach

1 cup frozen peas

1. Bring a large pot of water to a boil and cook the pasta according to package directions.

2. While the pasta is cooking, in a large sauté pan or skillet, heat the oil on medium-high heat. Add the nutritional yeast, red pepper flakes, garlic powder, onion powder, salt, and black pepper and cook for

about 2 minutes, until fragrant.

3. Add the tomato paste and vegetable broth and cook, stirring, for 3 minutes. Add the coconut milk and stir to form a sauce.

4. Drain the pasta, reserving ¼ cup of the pasta water. Add the spinach, peas, and pasta to the saucepan and toss to coat, adding the reserved pasta water, 2 tablespoons at a time, if needed to slightly loosen the sauce. Top with more nutritional yeast and serve.

PER SERVING: Calories: 336; Fat: 12g; Protein: 12g; Carbohydrates: 51g; Fiber: 8g

Curry Penne with Mango Chutney

PREP TIME: 5 minutes

COOK TIME: 15 minutes

EASY PREP, SOY-FREE

SERVES 4

Years ago, there was a popular upscale chain restaurant that we frequented that had a Madras curry penne dish on the menu. It was a complete departure from any type of pasta we'd had before, and my husband became hooked on it. This recipe is a play on that restaurant version, but with some vegetables added for extra color, texture, and nutritional value.

1 (16-ounce) box whole-wheat penne pasta

1 (13.5-ounce) can full-fat coconut milk

2 tablespoons Everyday Curry Paste or store-bought mild curry paste

2 cups frozen peas and carrots mix

2 tablespoons Mango Chutney or store-bought mango chutney

½ Granny Smith apple, cored and sliced into matchsticks

½ cup dried cranberries

1. Bring a large pot of water to a boil and cook the pasta according to package directions.

2. While the pasta is cooking, in a large sauté pan or skillet, combine the coconut milk and curry paste over medium-high heat and stir to form a sauce. Simmer on medium heat for 5 to 7 minutes, until the sauce thickens slightly.

3. Drain the pasta, reserving ¼ cup of the pasta water.

4. Add the pasta to the pan, along with the peas and carrots and chutney. Toss to coat. If the sauce is too thick, add the reserved pasta water to loosen it a bit.

5. Remove from the heat, add the apples and cranberries, and toss to

combine. Serve immediately.

PER SERVING: Calories: 693; Fat: 22g; Protein: 20g; Carbohydrates: 118g; Fiber: 16g

Burst Cherry Tomato Rigatoni

PREP TIME: 5 minutes

COOK TIME: 15 minutes

EASY PREP, NUT-FREE, SOY-FREE

SERVES 4

This is a great dish when farmers' markets are bursting with fresh tomatoes, but if you find yourself craving it midwinter, canned whole cherry tomatoes work as well; just reduce your cooking time slightly (since canned cherry tomatoes are softer than fresh).

1 (16-ounce) box whole-wheat rigatoni or similar tube-shaped pasta

3 tablespoons grapeseed or extra-virgin olive oil

4 garlic cloves, thinly sliced

Grated zest of ½ lemon

½ teaspoon red pepper

flakes ¼ teaspoon salt

3 pints whole cherry tomatoes or 3 (14-ounce) cans whole cherry

tomatoes ¼ cup chopped fresh basil

3 tablespoons nutritional yeast or vegan Parmesan cheese

1. Bring a large pot of water to a boil and cook the pasta according to package directions.

2. While the pasta is cooking, in a large sauté pan or skillet, heat the oil over medium heat. Add the garlic, lemon zest, red pepper flakes, and salt. Cook, stirring the garlic constantly, until it starts to lightly brown.

3. Add the cherry tomatoes (including the liquid if using canned) and reduce the heat to low. Cook until the tomatoes blister and soften, about 6 minutes. Use a fork or potato masher to gently mash about one-third of the tomatoes.

4. Drain the pasta, reserving 1 cup of pasta water. Add the pasta to the pan, along with ¼ cup of the pasta water, and toss. Continue adding the pasta water, in ¼-cup increments, until all the pasta is coated (it's okay if you don't use all the water). Top with the basil and nutritional yeast and serve.

VARY IT: Elevate this dish by adding zucchini slices and chopped onions to the pan with the garlic, or by crumbling in some mild Italian vegan sausage, such as Beyond Sausage, and cooking it with the garlic. Store-bought vegan sausage often contains coconut and other oils, so if using, eliminate or reduce the amount of oil called for.

PER SERVING: Calories: 555; Fat: 14g; Protein: 22g; Carbohydrates: 104g; Fiber: 15g

Pasta Primavera

PREP TIME: 15 minutes

COOK TIME: 15 minutes

NUT-FREE, SOY-FREE

SERVES 6

This is definitely a "vegetables first" type of dish, and it's one of my favorites. "Primavera" means springtime in Italian, and this recipe is a great way to showcase all the fresh spring and summer produce available. The key to preparing this dish in 30 minutes is to keep your vegetables the same size so they all cook evenly and quickly.

1 (16-ounce) box farfalle (bowtie) pasta

2 cups small broccoli florets

2 tablespoons grapeseed or extra-virgin olive oil

1 medium zucchini, halved lengthwise and cut into half moons

1 medium yellow summer squash, halved lengthwise and cut into half moons

1 red bell pepper, cut into matchsticks

½ medium red onion, thinly sliced

½ cup shredded carrots

1 cup grape tomatoes, halved

¼ cup water

½ vegan chicken or vegetable bouillon cube, crumbled 1 teaspoon minced garlic

1 cup fresh or frozen peas

¼ cup nutritional yeast or vegan Parmesan cheese

1. Bring a large pot of water to a boil and cook the pasta according to package directions. During the last 2 minutes of cooking, add the broccoli florets to the pasta. Drain, reserving ½ cup of the pasta water.

2. While the pasta is cooking, in a large sauté pan or skillet, heat the oil

on medium-high heat. Add the zucchini, summer squash, bell pepper, onion, and carrots. Cook for about 7 minutes, stirring frequently, until softened. Add the tomatoes, water, crumbled bouillon cube, and garlic. Cook for 2 minutes, or until the bouillon is dissolved.

3. Add the pasta and broccoli to the pan and toss to combine. Stir in the peas and nutritional yeast and cook for 2 to 3 minutes, until heated through. Serve.

SMART SHOPPING: To save prep time, look for precut fresh veggies in your grocer's produce department. Many grocery stores offer stir-fry kits that combine precut versions of many of the vegetables used in this dish.

PER SERVING: Calories: 399; Fat: 6g; Protein: 16g; Carbohydrates: 71g; Fiber: 7g

Creamy Sun-Dried Tomato and Spinach Pasta

PREP TIME: 5 minutes

COOK TIME: 20 minutes

EASY PREP, SOY-FREE

SERVES 6

I love serving this dish on busy weeknights. It's on the table in less than 30 minutes but tastes like it's been simmering all day. Sun-dried tomatoes add a deep, rich flavor to this dish and pair well with the creamy sauce. Be sure to use full-fat coconut milk here. Light versions have most of the fat removed and replaced with water, which will make your sauce too runny.

1 (16-ounce) box penne pasta

2 tablespoons grapeseed or olive oil

½ (8-ounce) jar oil-packed sun-dried tomatoes, drained and coarsely chopped

½ small onion, diced

1 teaspoon minced garlic

2 cups baby spinach

1 (13.5-ounce) can full-fat coconut milk

½ cup nutritional yeast

½ teaspoon Italian seasoning

½ teaspoon salt

½ teaspoon freshly ground black pepper

1. Bring a large pot of water to a boil and cook the pasta according to package instructions. Drain and set aside.

2. While the pasta is cooking, in a large sauté pan or skillet, heat the oil on medium-high heat. Add the tomatoes, onion, and garlic and cook for 5 minutes, until the onion is softened. Add the spinach and cook until the spinach is wilted, about 3 minutes.

3. Add the coconut milk to the skillet, lower the heat to medium, and let simmer for 10 minutes so the sauce can reduce slightly. Stir in the

nutritional yeast, Italian seasoning, salt, and pepper.

4. Add the pasta, toss to combine with the sauce, and serve.

VARY IT: Adding sliced mushrooms to this dish can boost that earthy, umami flavor. I like to use sliced mushrooms from the grocery store to save prep time. They are also a great replacement for sun-dried tomatoes along with a small amount of tomato paste.

PER SERVING: Calories: 516; Fat: 20g; Protein: 18g; Carbohydrates: 69g; Fiber: 7g

Vegetable Lo Mein

PREP TIME: 10 minutes

COOK TIME: 15 minutes

NUT-FREE

SERVES 4

This is a classic lo mein recipe with a vegan twist. Lo mein is typically made with egg noodles, so here I swap them out for whole-wheat spaghettini. There are eggless versions of lo mein noodles available, so if you're able to source them, feel free to use them instead. Customize this dish with whatever vegetables you have in your refrigerator.

8 ounces whole-wheat spaghettini or eggless lo mein noodles

2 cups broccoli florets

1 tablespoon mirin (Japanese cooking wine) or rice vinegar

1 tablespoon tamari

2 teaspoons sesame oil

1 teaspoon brown sugar or maple syrup

1 tablespoon grapeseed or extra-virgin olive oil

1 cup shredded carrots

1 green bell pepper, cut into strips

2 celery stalks, sliced diagonally

4 scallions, both white and green parts, chopped and divided

1 teaspoon minced garlic

4 cups bean sprouts

1 (8-ounce) can sliced water chestnuts, drained

1. Bring a large pot of water to a boil and cook the pasta according to package directions. During the last 2 minutes of cooking, add the broccoli. Drain and set aside.

2. While the pasta is cooking, in a small bowl, whisk the mirin, tamari, sesame oil, and brown sugar together.

3. In a large sauté pan or skillet, heat the grapeseed oil on medium-high heat. Add the carrots, bell pepper, celery, white parts of the scallions, and garlic and cook for about 5 minutes, until the vegetables are soft.

4. Add the noodles, broccoli, bean sprouts, water chestnuts, and sauce and cook, tossing to combine, for 3 minutes, or until all the sauce is absorbed. Sprinkle with the green scallions and serve.

VARY IT: Try adding some crispy pan-fried tofu to this dish or pairing it with the Sweet and Spicy Tofu with Green Beans, Orange Tofu, or Fiery Tofu with Cashews for an authentic "better than takeout" experience.

INGREDIENT TIP: If you have Stir-Fry Sauce on hand, you can substitute ¼ cup of it for the mirin-tamari sauce.

PER SERVING: Calories: 361; Fat: 7g; Protein: 13g; Carbohydrates: 63g; Fiber: 8g

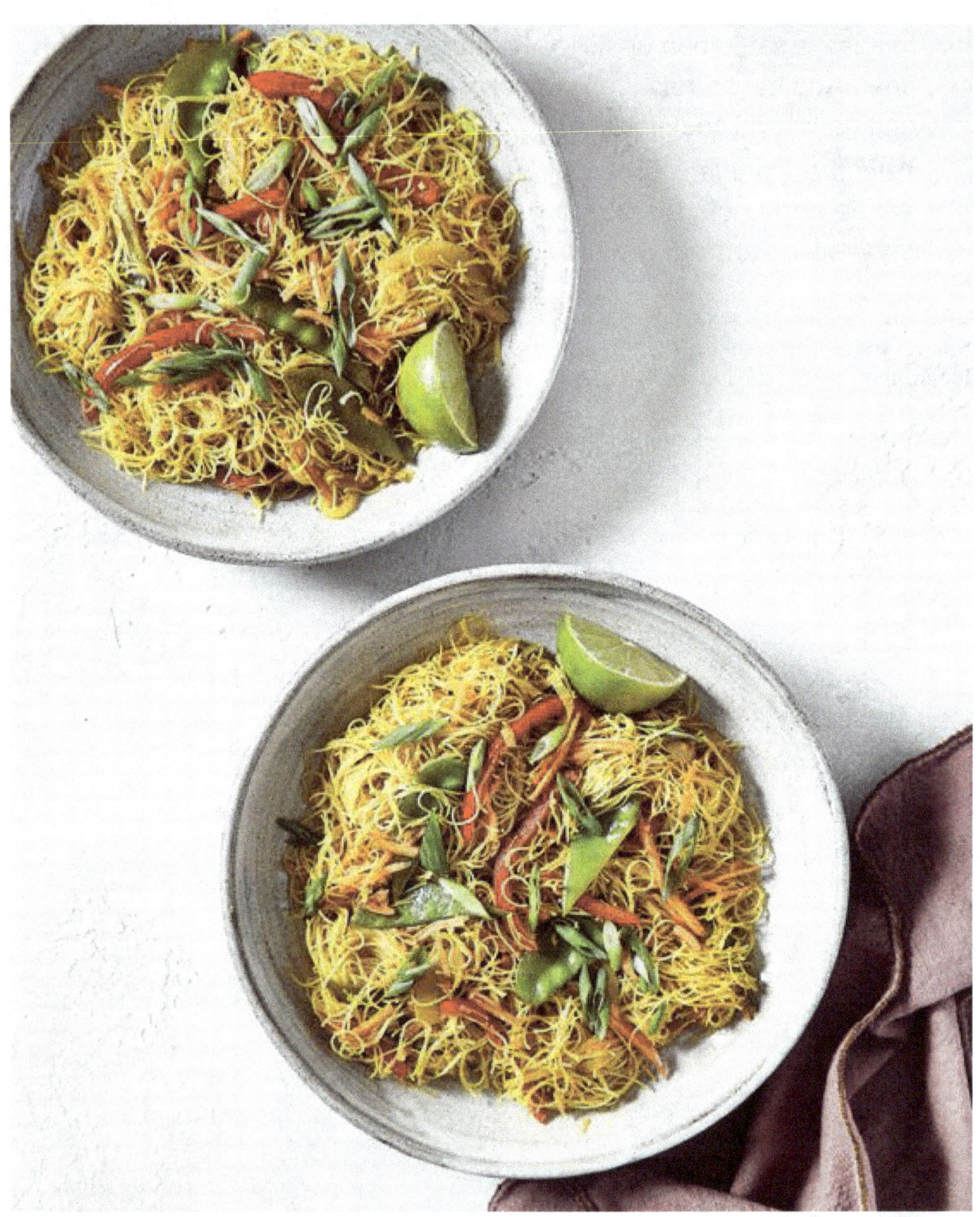

Singapore-Style Vermicelli

PREP TIME: 10 minutes

COOK TIME: 10 minutes

NUT-FREE

SERVES 4

This is one of my favorite "better than takeout" dishes. It's on the table in less time than your local delivery service's version, and it's just as delicious. I like to make this at the end of a week when I've got stray, leftover veggies in the refrigerator to use up. You can add almost any vegetable here. Because this dish cooks so quickly, steam large vegetables like broccoli or cauliflower before adding to the pan.

1 (14-ounce) package rice vermicelli noodles

1 cup water

¼ cup low-sodium soy

sauce 1 teaspoon sugar

2 tablespoons grapeseed or extra-virgin olive

oil ½ medium onion, sliced

½ red bell pepper,

sliced ½ carrot, grated

1 cup snow peas, halved

1 teaspoon minced garlic

1 teaspoon grated ginger

1 tablespoon mild curry powder

2 scallions, green part only, chopped, for garnish

1 lime, quartered, for garnish

1. Cook the noodles according to package directions. Drain and rinse under cold water. Set aside.

2. While the noodles are soaking, in a small bowl, whisk the water, soy sauce, and sugar.

3. In a large sauté pan or skillet, heat the oil over medium-high heat. Add the onion, bell pepper, and carrot and cook for about 4 minutes, until the vegetables are soft. Add the snow peas, garlic, and ginger and cook, stirring constantly, for 1 minute, until fragrant.

4. Add the vermicelli noodles and curry powder and toss to coat. Reduce the heat to medium. Add the prepared sauce and simmer, tossing occasionally, until the liquid is absorbed, about 4 minutes. Garnish with scallions and lime wedges to serve.

VARY IT: Boost the protein in this dish by adding some pan-fried tofu cubes or Korean Barbecue– Style Tofu.

PER SERVING: Calories: 461; Fat: 9g; Protein: 8g; Carbohydrates: 89g; Fiber: 5g

Udon Noodles with Mushrooms and Cabbage

PREP TIME: 10 minutes

COOK TIME: 10 minutes

NUT-FREE

SERVES 4

This dish is based on a very popular Chinese dish, Shanghai fried noodles, which typically combines thick, long egg noodles, meat, and vegetables in a light, savory, sweet sauce. I give this dish a plant-based twist by using Japanese udon noodles to mimic the shape and consistency of the Shanghai fried noodles and adding a ton of vegetables. Using precut vegetables from your grocer's fresh produce section saves prep time and enables you to cook this dish in only a few minutes.

1 (16-ounce) package udon noodles

2 tablespoons grapeseed or extra-virgin olive oil

2 cups sliced cremini mushrooms

1 zucchini, halved lengthwise and cut into half moons

1 red bell pepper, chopped

½ medium onion, chopped

3 scallions, white and green parts, chopped and

divided ½ head napa cabbage, shredded

⅓ cup hoisin sauce or Stir-Fry Sauce

1. Cook the udon noodles according to package directions.

2. While the noodles are cooking, in a large sauté pan or skillet, heat the oil on high heat. Add the mushrooms, zucchini, red pepper, onion, and white parts of the scallions and cook, stirring constantly, for 5 minutes, or until the vegetables soften and are a bit charred or dark.

3. Reduce the heat to medium-high, add the cabbage, and cook for 1 minute, until heated through.

4. Drain the noodles and add to the vegetables. Add the hoisin sauce, toss to coat, and serve.

STRETCH IT: Stretch this dish even further by adding some baked or pan-fried tofu or store-bought vegan "beef."

PER SERVING: Calories: 536; Fat: 11g; Protein: 20g; Carbohydrates: 94g; Fiber: 10g

Creamy Cajun Mushroom Pasta

PREP TIME: 5 minutes

COOK TIME: 20 minutes

EASY PREP, SOY-FREE

SERVES 6

I have a daughter who loves mushrooms, and this dish has become one of her favorites. I like it because I can get it on the table in under 30 minutes, making it a great "busy night" dinner. My trick is buying presliced mushrooms, which saves a ton of prep time. If you're not a fan of spicy dishes, swap out the Cajun seasoning for dried oregano and thyme.

1 (16-ounce) box whole-wheat fusilli pasta

1 tablespoon grapeseed or extra-virgin olive oil

1 tablespoon vegan butter

1 pound sliced cremini or baby bella mushrooms

½ medium onion, diced

1 (13.5-ounce) can full-fat coconut milk

½ cup low-sodium vegetable

broth ¼ cup nutritional yeast

1 tablespoon Cajun seasoning

2 tablespoons chopped fresh parsley or 1 tablespoon dried parsley, for garnish

1. Bring a large pot of water to a boil and cook the pasta according to package directions. Drain and set aside.

2. While the pasta is cooking, in a large sauté pan or skillet, heat the oil and butter on medium-high heat. Add the mushrooms and onion and cook for about 6 minutes, until the mushrooms are softened.

3. Add the coconut milk, vegetable broth, nutritional yeast, and Cajun seasoning and stir to combine. Reduce the heat to medium and simmer for 10 minutes, or until the sauce thickens enough to coat the back of a spoon.

4. Add the pasta and toss to combine. Sprinkle the parsley on top and serve.

INGREDIENT TIP: If you can't find Cajun seasoning, make your own by combining 3 tablespoons smoked paprika, 2 tablespoons kosher salt, 2 tablespoons garlic powder, 1 tablespoon ground black pepper, 1 tablespoon onion powder, 1 tablespoon dried oregano, 1 tablespoon cayenne pepper, and ½ teaspoon dried thyme. Store the leftovers in an airtight jar in your spice rack.

PER SERVING: Calories: 468; Fat: 17g; Protein: 16g; Carbohydrates: 66g; Fiber: 5g

6

Stir-Fries and Curries

Broccoli Ramen Stir-Fry
Sweet and Spicy Tofu with Green Beans
Butter Bean Kurma
Fiery Tofu with Cashews
Vegetable Fried Rice
Red Curry Vegetables
Cauliflower, Potato, and Pea Curry
Orange Tofu
Wicked Hot Clean-Out-the-Fridge Curry
Curried Okra and Tomatoes
Kung Pao Broccoli and Cauliflower
Egg-Roll-in-a-Bowl Stir-Fry
Eat-the-Rainbow Vegetable Stir-Fry
Coconut Curry Ramen
Sweet Potato and Spinach Curry
Butter Chicken Tofu
Yellow Curried Chickpeas with Kale

Stir-Fried Teriyaki Udon Bowl

Broccoli Ramen Stir-Fry

PREP TIME: 15 minutes

COOK TIME: 10 minutes

NUT-FREE

SERVES 4

I always keep a few packages of ramen noodles in my pantry for quick lunches or weeknight dinners. They make an excellent base for stir-fries and soups. If you have access to an Asian supermarket in your neighborhood, you can buy bags of just the noodles, but if not, grab any kind from your supermarket—we're discarding the seasoning packets and making our own healthier, more flavorful sauce for this dish.

For the sauce

¼ cup low-sodium soy sauce

1 tablespoon cornstarch

⅓ cup low-sodium vegetable broth

2 tablespoons hoisin sauce

1 tablespoon maple syrup

1 tablespoon rice vinegar

1 tablespoon sesame oil

1½ teaspoons grated ginger

¼ to ½ teaspoon sriracha or other hot sauce

For the stir-fry

2 (3-ounce) packages ramen noodles (seasoning packets discarded)

3 cups broccoli florets

1 tablespoon grapeseed or extra-virgin olive oil

1 yellow bell pepper, thinly sliced

1 cup shredded carrots

½ medium onion, thinly sliced

Sesame seeds, for garnish

1. To make the sauce: In a small bowl, whisk together the soy sauce and cornstarch until no lumps remain. Add the vegetable broth, hoisin sauce, maple syrup, rice vinegar, sesame oil, ginger, and sriracha and whisk until smooth.

2. Bring a large pot of water to a boil and cook the ramen noodles and broccoli together for 2 to 3 minutes, or until the noodles are just tender. Drain and rinse under cold water. Set aside.

3. In a large sauté pan or skillet, heat the grapeseed oil on medium-high heat. Add the bell pepper, carrots, and onion and cook for about 5 minutes, until the onion is just tender and translucent.

4. Add the cooked noodles, broccoli, and sauce. Using tongs, toss everything together and cook for about 2 minutes, until coated and warmed through. Garnish with sesame seeds and serve.

INGREDIENT TIP: If you have homemade Stir-Fry Sauce on hand, use 1 cup of that in place of the sauce here.

PER SERVING: Calories: 342; Fat: 15g; Protein: 8g; Carbohydrates: 45g; Fiber: 4g

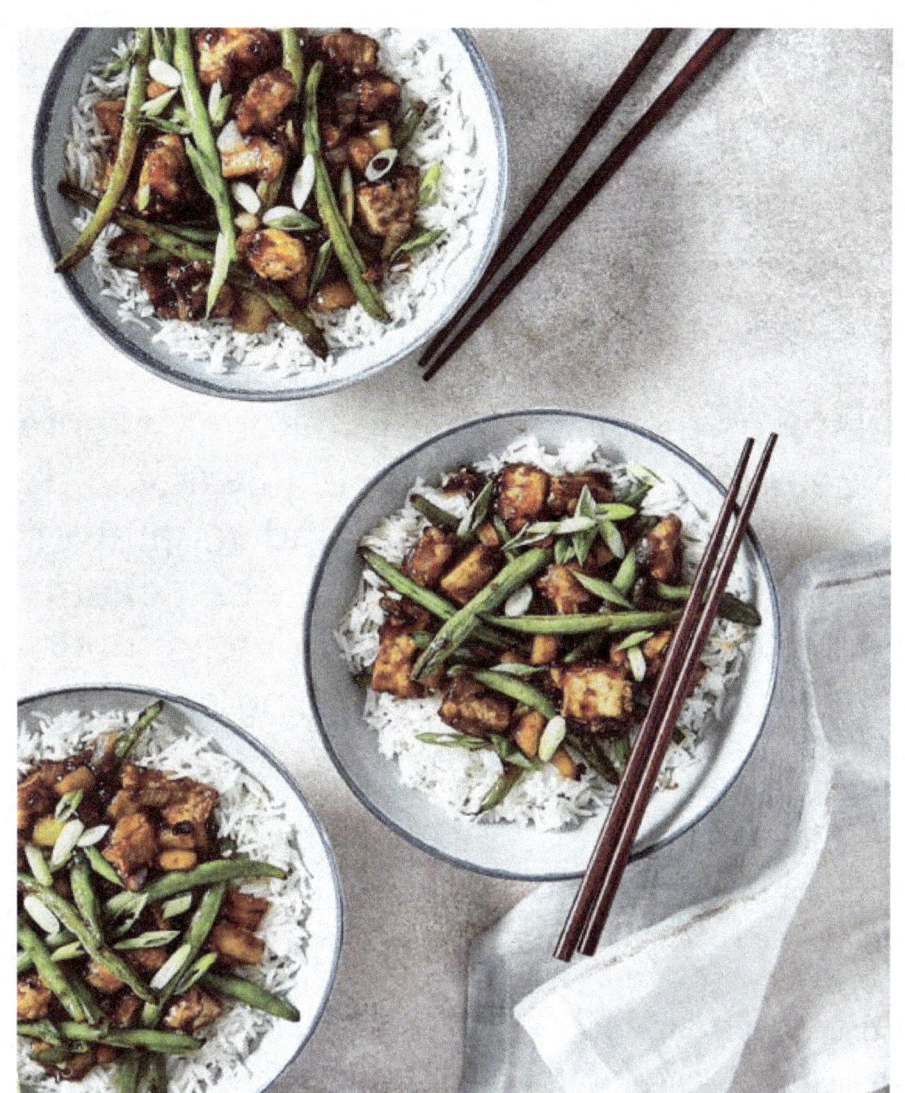

Sweet and Spicy Tofu with Green Beans

PREP TIME: 10 minutes

COOK TIME: 15 minutes

GLUTEN-FREE, NUT-FREE

SERVES 4

This dish reminds me of an all-time takeout favorite of ours: Szechuan beef. This version has a boldly flavored, sticky sauce that coats the chunks of tofu and vegetables when cooked at a high heat to give them a sweet, charred flavor. I like to rip the tofu for this dish to expose its rough edges (the uneven edges are great for catching sauce), but you can just cube the tofu if you prefer.

2¼ cups water, divided

1 cup jasmine or basmati rice, rinsed

2 tablespoons grapeseed or extra-virgin olive oil, divided

8 ounces green beans

1 medium onion, chopped

1 bell pepper, chopped

1 (14-ounce) block extra-firm tofu, ripped into small chunks

½ teaspoon grated ginger

1 teaspoon minced garlic

½ cup tamari

¼ cup packed brown sugar

2 tablespoons cornstarch

½ to 1 teaspoon sriracha

2 scallions, both green and white parts, chopped

1. In a medium pot, bring 2 cups of water to a boil. Add the rice, cover, and reduce the heat to low. Cook for 15 minutes, then remove from the heat, keeping the lid on.

2. While the rice is cooking, in a large sauté pan or skillet, heat 1

tablespoon of oil over high heat. Add the green beans, onion, and bell pepper and cook for about 4 minutes, until the vegetables are lightly charred and softened. Remove them from the pan and set aside.

3. Add the remaining 1 tablespoon of oil to the pan and lower the heat to medium-high. Add the tofu and cook for about 5 minutes, until golden and crispy on all sides. Return the vegetables to the pan, along with the garlic and ginger, and cook for 2 minutes while you make the sauce.

4. In a small bowl, whisk together the tamari, remaining ¼ cup of water, brown sugar, cornstarch, and sriracha. Pour the sauce into the pan, tossing the tofu and vegetables with it. Cook for 2 to 3 minutes, or until the sauce thickens and coats the tofu. Sprinkle with the scallions and serve over the rice.

VARY IT: Try serving this dish over cooked quinoa instead of rice. Quinoa is gluten-free and is a powerhouse of nutrition with twice the fiber and protein of rice.

PER SERVING: Calories: 452; Fat: 13g; Protein: 19g; Carbohydrates: 67g; Fiber: 5g

Butter Bean Kurma

PREP TIME: 5 minutes

COOK TIME: 20 minutes

EASY PREP, GLUTEN-FREE, NUT-FREE, ONE POT, SOY-FREE

SERVES 4

This recipe is inspired by a friend's homemade version we tasted a few years ago. That one was made with dried beans soaked overnight and a long, slow cooking process. I created a 30-minute version to serve when I'm in the mood for good food in a hurry. I like to serve it on basmati rice, which takes just 15 minutes to make and can cook right alongside this dish.

2 tablespoons extra-virgin olive oil or grapeseed oil

1 small onion, diced

1 teaspoon minced garlic

1 teaspoon ground cumin

1 teaspoon ground turmeric

1 teaspoon chili powder

½ teaspoon ground cinnamon

½ teaspoon salt

1 (15-ounce) can diced tomatoes

1 (15-ounce) can butter beans, drained and rinsed

1 tablespoon freshly squeezed lime juice

1 tablespoon brown sugar

1. In a large sauté pan or skillet, heat the oil on medium-high heat. Add the onion and cook for 3 minutes, until softened. Add the garlic, cumin, turmeric, chili powder, cinnamon, and salt and stir to combine.

2. Reduce the heat to medium. Add the tomatoes and their juices, butter beans, lime juice, and brown sugar and cook for 12 to 15 minutes, or until the tomatoes and beans are soft. Serve over rice or naan.

INGREDIENT TIP: Butter beans are large, flat, chewy beans named for their resemblance in color and richness to a common dairy staple. Sold in cans at most grocery stores, butter beans are packed with fiber and protein and are low in fat.

PER SERVING: Calories: 198; Fat: 8g; Protein: 6g; Carbohydrates: 27g; Fiber: 9g

Fiery Tofu with Cashews

PREP TIME: 10 minutes

COOK TIME: 15 minutes

SERVES 3

This dish is fiery-hot and slightly sweet and has quickly become a favorite dish in our house. If I'm making it for my kids, I'll dial down the hot sauce a bit (and serve it on noodles or rice), but if I'm the only one dining it's full steam ahead on heat. This dish pairs really well with garlicky steamed broccoli or sautéed bok choy with garlic and soy sauce if you're looking for a low-carb side dish.

1 cup freshly squeezed orange juice (from 3 to 4 oranges) or store-bought pulp-free orange juice

½ cup sweet Thai chili

sauce Juice of 2 lemons

3 tablespoons low-sodium soy sauce

2 tablespoons sriracha

½ teaspoon plus ⅓ cup cornstarch, divided

2 tablespoons grapeseed or extra-virgin olive oil

1 (14-ounce) block extra-firm tofu, drained, pressed, and cut into 1-inch cubes

1 cup roasted unsalted cashews

3 scallions, green part only, finely chopped

1. In a medium bowl, combine the orange juice, Thai chili sauce, lemon juice, soy sauce, sriracha, and ½ teaspoon of cornstarch. Whisk to combine. Set aside.

2. In a large sauté pan or skillet, heat the oil on medium-high heat. In a large resealable bag, toss the tofu and remaining ⅓ cup of cornstarch together. Shake well to coat the tofu, then add to the hot pan and cook for 8 to 10 minutes, until the tofu is golden and crisp on all sides.

3. Add the sauce to the pan and simmer until thick, tossing the tofu to

coat it, about 5 minutes. Add the cashews and scallions and serve.

DIETARY TIP: Want to make this dish oil-free? Skip the pan-fry (and the cornstarch coating) and bake the tofu instead. Preheat the oven to 400°F and line a rimmed baking sheet with parchment paper. Arrange the cut tofu on the prepared baking sheet in a single layer and bake for 20 minutes, tossing the pieces halfway through. Heat the sauce as above and add the baked tofu to it just before serving.

PER SERVING: Calories: 671; Fat: 35g; Protein: 25g; Carbohydrates: 60g; Fiber: 8g

Vegetable Fried Rice

PREP TIME: 10 minutes

COOK TIME: 15 minutes

NUT-FREE

SERVES 4

Fried rice is a great "use up what's in the fridge" meal. I have this habit of always cooking too much rice, and this is a great way to put those leftovers to use. Of course, you can also make this dish in the time it takes to cook a pot of rice. The trick is to use small frozen vegetables, like peas, carrots, and green beans, that can warm up in a couple of minutes.

¼ cup low-sodium soy
sauce 1 teaspoon sugar

½ teaspoon sesame oil

2 cups low-sodium vegetable broth

1 cup basmati rice, rinsed

1 tablespoon grapeseed or extra-virgin olive oil

1 small onion, diced

1 cup chopped mushrooms

3 scallions, both white and green parts, chopped and divided

2 cups frozen mixed vegetables (peas, carrots, corn, green or wax beans)

1. In a small bowl, combine the soy sauce, sugar, and sesame oil. Set aside.

2. In a medium pot with a tight-fitting lid, combine the vegetable broth and rice and bring to a boil. Immediately reduce the heat to low and cook, covered, for 15 minutes. Remove from the heat, fluff with a fork, and set aside.

3. While the rice is cooking, heat the grapeseed oil on medium-high heat. Add the onion, mushrooms, and white parts of the scallions and cook for about 6 minutes, until the onion is translucent and the

mushrooms are softened.

4. Add the cooked rice and frozen vegetables and cook for 1 minute, or until the vegetables are warmed through, tossing to combine. Pour in the sauce and toss to coat the rice.

5. Sprinkle with the green scallions and serve.

PER SERVING: Calories: 287; Fat: 5g; Protein: 8g; Carbohydrates: 54g; Fiber: 5g

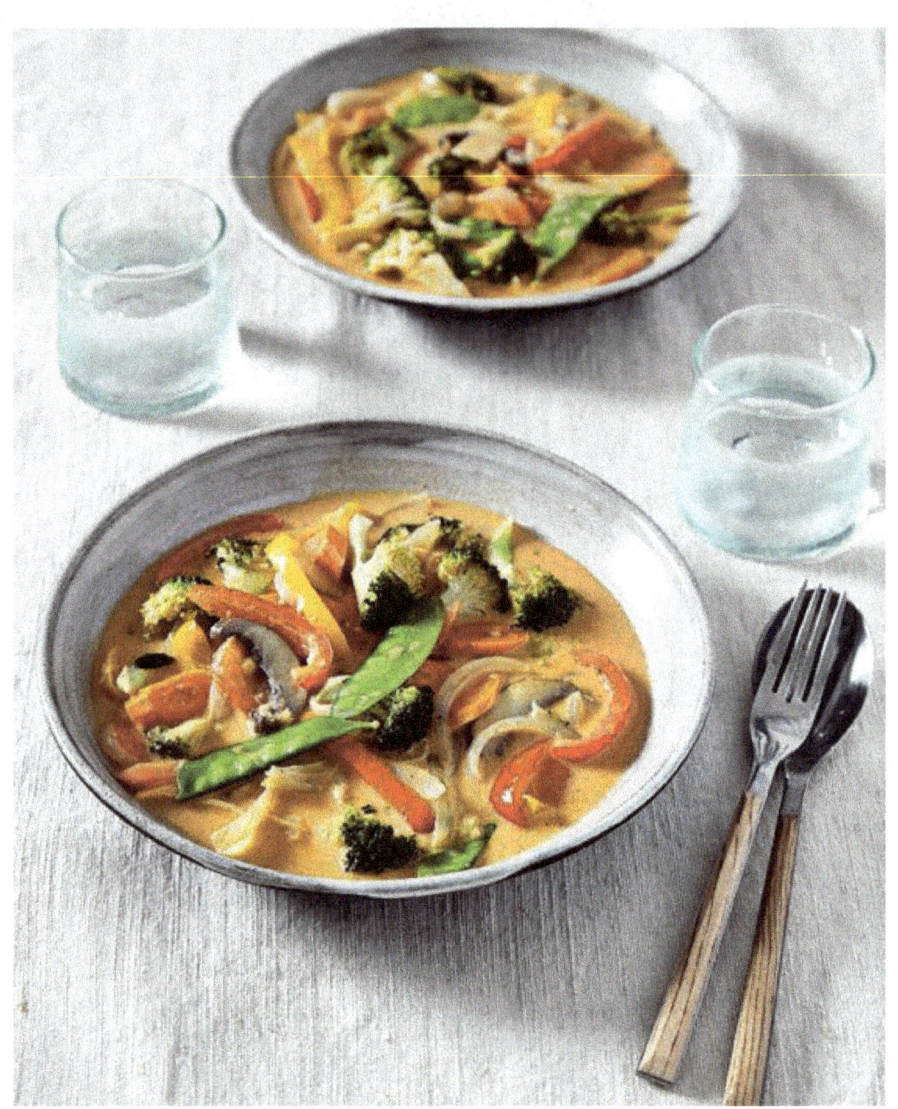

Red Curry Vegetables

PREP TIME: 5 minutes

COOK TIME: 15 minutes

EASY PREP, GLUTEN-FREE, SOY-FREE

SERVES 3

This dish is healthier than takeout! Use frozen stir-fry vegetable mixes in this dish to add a variety of vegetables and reduce prep time. I like serving this over homemade coconut rice, which you can easily make by using a regular jasmine rice recipe and swapping 1 cup of water for 1 cup of full-fat coconut milk plus 1 tablespoon of sugar.

1 tablespoon grapeseed or extra-virgin olive oil

1 medium onion, diced

1 teaspoon minced garlic

1 teaspoon grated ginger

1 (12-ounce) bag frozen stir-fry vegetables

1 (13.5-ounce) can full-fat coconut milk

½ cup low-sodium vegetable broth

1 tablespoon Thai red curry paste 2

teaspoons cold water

1 teaspoon cornstarch

1. In a large sauté pan or skillet, heat the oil on medium-high heat. Add the onion and cook for about 5 minutes, until translucent. Add the garlic and ginger and cook, stirring constantly, for 30 seconds, until fragrant. Add the frozen vegetables and stir to combine.

2. Pour in the coconut milk, vegetable broth, and curry paste and bring to a simmer. Cook for 7 to 10 minutes, until the vegetables are fork-tender.

3. In a small bowl, mix the water and cornstarch. Add the cornstarch slurry to the pan and stir continuously for 1 minute, or until the sauce

thickens. Serve.

PER SERVING: Calories: 328; Fat: 27g; Protein: 5g; Carbohydrates: 20g; Fiber: 5g

Cauliflower, Potato, and Pea Curry

PREP TIME: 10 minutes

COOK TIME: 15 minutes

GLUTEN-FREE, SOY-FREE

SERVES 4

This dish is a take on aloo gobi, a traditional Indian curry made from cauliflower and potato. My version is a really easy curry that comes together in just minutes and incorporates other vegetables as well. The key to reducing prep time and getting this dish on the table in under 30 minutes is to use precut, bagged, or frozen vegetables. You can easily customize this dish by adding whatever vegetables you have in your refrigerator or freezer.

2 large yellow potatoes, diced

2 cups cauliflower florets

1 tablespoon grapeseed or extra-virgin olive oil

1 medium onion, diced

½ teaspoon minced garlic

2 cups frozen peas and carrots

2 tablespoons Everyday Curry Paste or store-bought mild curry paste

1 (13.5-ounce) can full-fat coconut milk

1. Bring a large pot of water to a boil and cook the potatoes and cauliflower for 8 to 10 minutes, until just fork-tender. Drain and set aside.

2. While the potatoes and cauliflower are cooking, in a large sauté pan or skillet, heat the oil on medium-high heat. Add the onion and cook until just translucent, about 4 minutes. Add the garlic and cook for 30 seconds, until fragrant.

3. Add the peas and carrots and curry paste and stir to combine. Pour in

the coconut milk and simmer until the sauce thickens slightly. Add the cooked potatoes and cauliflower, stirring to coat. Serve.

PER SERVING: Calories: 390; Fat: 22g; Protein: 8g; Carbohydrates: 47g; Fiber: 9g

Orange Tofu

PREP TIME: 10 minutes

COOK TIME: 15 minutes

NUT-FREE

SERVES 4

This is a dish that will keep you from reaching for the takeout menu or opening up that delivery app on your phone. In the time it would take you to get delivery, you can whip up this dish. I like to pair it with Vegetable Lo Mein or Vegetable Fried Rice for the full better-than-takeout experience.

1 cup freshly squeezed orange juice (from 3 to 4 oranges)

3 tablespoons grated orange zest (from 1 orange)

½ cup sugar

2 tablespoons rice or white wine vinegar

2 tablespoons low-sodium soy sauce

¼ teaspoon minced garlic

¼ teaspoon grated ginger

¼ teaspoon red pepper flakes

4 tablespoons cornstarch, divided

1 tablespoon grapeseed or extra-virgin olive oil

1 (14-ounce) block extra-firm tofu, drained, pressed, and cut into 1-inch cubes

2 scallions, green part only, chopped

1. In a medium saucepan, combine the orange juice and zest, sugar, vinegar, soy sauce, garlic, ginger, red pepper flakes, and 1 tablespoon of cornstarch. Bring to a boil and simmer for about 3 minutes until thickened, stirring constantly. Remove from the heat and set aside.

2. In a large sauté pan or skillet, heat the oil on medium-high heat. In a large resealable bag, toss the tofu and remaining 3 tablespoons of cornstarch together. Shake well to coat the tofu, then add to the hot pan and cook for 8 to 10 minutes, until the tofu is golden and crisp on

all sides.

3. Add the sauce to the pan and toss the tofu to coat it. Sprinkle with the scallions and serve.

DIETARY TIP: Lower the soy content in this dish by swapping the tofu for cauliflower. Cut 1 head of cauliflower into florets, drizzle with olive oil, salt, and pepper, and bake at 400°F for 15 to 20 minutes, or until lightly golden and fork tender. Toss with the orange sauce and garnish with the scallions, then serve.

PER SERVING: Calories: 302; Fat: 9g; Protein: 12g; Carbohydrates: 44g; Fiber: 2g

Wicked Hot Clean-Out-the-Fridge Curry

PREP TIME: 10 minutes

COOK TIME: 20 minutes

GLUTEN-FREE, SOY-FREE

SERVES 4

It feels funny writing this one out as a recipe, since I basically took whatever half-used or about-to-expire vegetables I had laying around one day, cooked them up in a really fragrant and spicy curry sauce, and called it dinner. The recipe below is based on the leftover veggies I usually have on hand, but you can swap out or add to it based on what's occupying space in your refrigerator.

1 (12-ounce) bag fresh or frozen mixed broccoli, cauliflower, and carrots

2 to 3 tablespoons water

1 tablespoon grapeseed or extra-virgin olive oil

1 large zucchini, chopped

4 or 5 cremini or white button mushrooms, stems removed and caps sliced

1 medium onion, diced

1 pint cherry or grape tomatoes

1 bell pepper, chopped

1 heaping tablespoon store-bought vindaloo curry paste, or 1 heaping tablespoon Everyday Curry Paste plus 1 teaspoon sriracha

1 (13.5-ounce) can full-fat coconut milk

½ cup low-sodium vegetable broth

1. In a large microwaveable dish, combine the broccoli, cauliflower, and carrots with the water. Cover with a plate and microwave for 3 minutes, or until just tender when pierced with a fork.

2. While the vegetables are steaming, in a large sauté pan or skillet, heat the oil on medium-high heat and add the zucchini, mushrooms, and onion. Cook until the onion is translucent, about 5 minutes.

3. Add the tomatoes, bell pepper, steamed vegetables, and curry paste and cook for 2 minutes, stirring constantly, until the curry paste is fragrant and warmed through.

4. Pour in the coconut milk and vegetable broth and simmer over medium heat for 10 to 12 minutes, until all the vegetables are soft. Serve.

PER SERVING: Calories: 281; Fat: 21g; Protein: 6g; Carbohydrates: 22g; Fiber: 6g

Curried Okra and Tomatoes

PREP TIME: 5 minutes

COOK TIME: 15 minutes

EASY PREP, GLUTEN-FREE, NUT-FREE, SOY-FREE

SERVES 4

I based this recipe on a menu item from our favorite Indian restaurant. Since we are outside their delivery area now, when we get a craving for their bhindi masala, I whip this one up instead. I like to use frozen chopped okra because it saves time and turns this into a "20 minutes or less" dish. If you have a bag of frozen diced onions on hand, you can make this a 15-minute dinner.

1 tablespoon grapeseed or extra-virgin olive oil

1 (12-ounce) bag frozen chopped okra

1 medium onion, diced

1 (28-ounce) can diced tomatoes

2 tablespoons Everyday Curry Paste or store-bought mild curry paste

2 teaspoons cold water

1 teaspoon cornstarch

1. In a large sauté pan or skillet, heat the oil on medium-high heat. Add the okra and onion and cook for about 8 minutes, until the onion is just translucent and the okra is barely soft. Add the tomatoes and their juices and the curry paste and simmer for 5 minutes.

2. In a small bowl, mix the water and cornstarch together until smooth and add to the pan, stirring constantly for 1 minute, or until the sauce thickens enough to coat the back of a spoon. Serve.

INGREDIENT TIP: Also known as ladies' fingers, okra is a common vegetable in the United States, Africa, India, and the Caribbean. It's a nutritional powerhouse, known for its high levels of calcium, potassium, and vitamins A, C, and K. Okra pairs well with spicy preparations, such as gumbo or bhindi masala. You can find it at most grocery stores in the fresh produce section or frozen in bags in the frozen vegetable or international sections.

PER SERVING: Calories: 134; Fat: 5g; Protein: 4g; Carbohydrates: 20g; Fiber: 6g

Kung Pao Broccoli and Cauliflower

PREP TIME: 10 minutes

COOK TIME: 20 minutes

NUT-FREE

SERVES 4

This recipe gives you the flavor and texture of battered and fried kung pao, but with a healthier, baked twist. I like to use broccoli and cauliflower here because they are a switch from the standard tofu, and because they both hold up well to the breading, baking, and sauce. I've included a recipe for homemade kung pao sauce, but if you have a jarred version on hand, you may use that instead.

For the vegetables

1 tablespoon grapeseed or extra-virgin olive oil

1¼ cups unsweetened soy milk

1 cup all-purpose or chickpea flour

½ teaspoon salt

½ teaspoon baking powder

1 (12-ounce) bag mixed broccoli and cauliflower florets

For the sauce

½ cup low-sodium soy sauce

½ cup maple syrup

¼ cup rice vinegar

¼ cup cold water

2 tablespoons cornstarch

2 teaspoons sesame oil

2 teaspoons grated ginger

1 teaspoon minced garlic

1 teaspoon sriracha

1. Preheat the oven to 450°F. Line a rimmed baking sheet with parchment paper and brush with the grapeseed oil. Set aside.

2. In a large bowl, stir together the soy milk, flour, salt, and baking powder. Add the broccoli and cauliflower and toss to coat. Remove the florets and place them on the prepared baking sheet. Bake for 15 minutes, until lightly browned.

3. To make the sauce: While the vegetables bake, in a small saucepan whisk together the soy sauce, maple syrup, rice vinegar, water, cornstarch, sesame oil, ginger, garlic, and sriracha on medium heat and simmer for 8 to 10 minutes, or until the sauce is glossy and thick.

4. Remove the cooked broccoli and cauliflower florets from the oven and place in a large bowl. Pour the sauce over the florets and toss to coat.

DIETARY TIP: If you're not a fan of breading, or you are gluten-free, you can simply roast the broccoli and cauliflower with a little bit of olive oil, salt, and pepper for 15 minutes and then toss with the sauce.

PER SERVING: Calories: 352; Fat: 7g; Protein: 10g; Carbohydrates: 61g; Fiber: 4g

Egg-Roll-in-a-Bowl Stir-Fry

PREP TIME: 5 minutes

COOK TIME: 15 minutes

EASY PREP, NUT-FREE

SERVES 4

This dish has all the classic flavors of an egg roll, but without the deep-frying or the wrapper. It's delicious as a meal on its own or as a filling for lettuce wraps. I've used tempeh to add protein, but you could swap it out for tofu if you prefer. You could also add some slivered snow peas or water chestnuts for more crunch.

2 tablespoons canola or grapeseed oil, divided

1 (7-ounce) package tempeh, crumbled

1 large onion, diced

1 (10-ounce) bag shredded cabbage

2 cups shredded carrots

¼ cup tamari or dark soy sauce

2 tablespoons sesame oil

1 tablespoon grated ginger

2 teaspoons minced garlic

½ teaspoon freshly ground black pepper

1. In a large sauté pan or skillet, heat 1 tablespoon of canola oil on medium-high heat. Add the tempeh and onion and cook for 4 minutes, until the onion is just translucent.

2. Reduce the heat to medium and add the cabbage and carrots. Cook for 4 minutes, stirring occasionally.

3. While the vegetables are cooking, in a small bowl, whisk together the tamari, sesame oil, ginger, garlic, pepper, and remaining 1 tablespoon of oil.

4. Pour the sauce over the cabbage mixture in the pan and toss well to coat. Continue cooking for 5 to 10 minutes, or until the cabbage is tender, and serve.

PER SERVING: Calories: 285; Fat: 19g; Protein: 14g; Carbohydrates: 18g; Fiber: 6g

Eat-the-Rainbow Vegetable Stir-Fry

PREP TIME: 5 minutes

COOK TIME: 15 minutes

EASY PREP, NUT-FREE

SERVES 3

This dish is all about the sauce. Teriyaki is a fabulous Japanese sauce and is delicious in almost any type of stir-fry. But store-bought brands can be full of sugar, salt, and preservatives. This recipe uses a homemade version that avoids excess salt and sugar but still adds a ton of flavor. For extra variety without extra prep, use bags of frozen stir-fry vegetables.

1 teaspoon grapeseed or extra-virgin olive oil
1 medium onion, diced
6 white button or cremini mushrooms, stems removed and caps sliced
1 (12-ounce) bag frozen Asian-style stir-fry vegetables
½ cup cold water
2 tablespoons low-sodium soy sauce
1 tablespoon brown sugar
2 teaspoons cornstarch
1 teaspoon maple syrup
¼ teaspoon grated ginger
¼ teaspoon garlic powder

1. In a large sauté pan or skillet, heat the oil on medium-high heat. Add the onion and mushrooms and cook for about 4 minutes, until the onion starts to soften. Add the frozen vegetables and cook for about 6 minutes, until almost tender.

2. In a small bowl, whisk together the water, soy sauce, brown sugar, cornstarch, maple syrup, ginger, and garlic powder until smooth. Pour into the pan with the vegetables and cook for 4 to 5 minutes, until the sauce thickens. Serve over quinoa, rice, or noodles.

STRETCH IT: Double or triple the batch of teriyaki sauce and use it for other meals. It works well with many other dishes in this book. Simply combine all the ingredients in a small pan and simmer on medium heat for 5 to 8 minutes, until glossy and thick. Store in an airtight jar in the refrigerator for up to a week.

PER SERVING: Calories: 107; Fat: 2g; Protein: 5g; Carbohydrates: 20g; Fiber: 4g

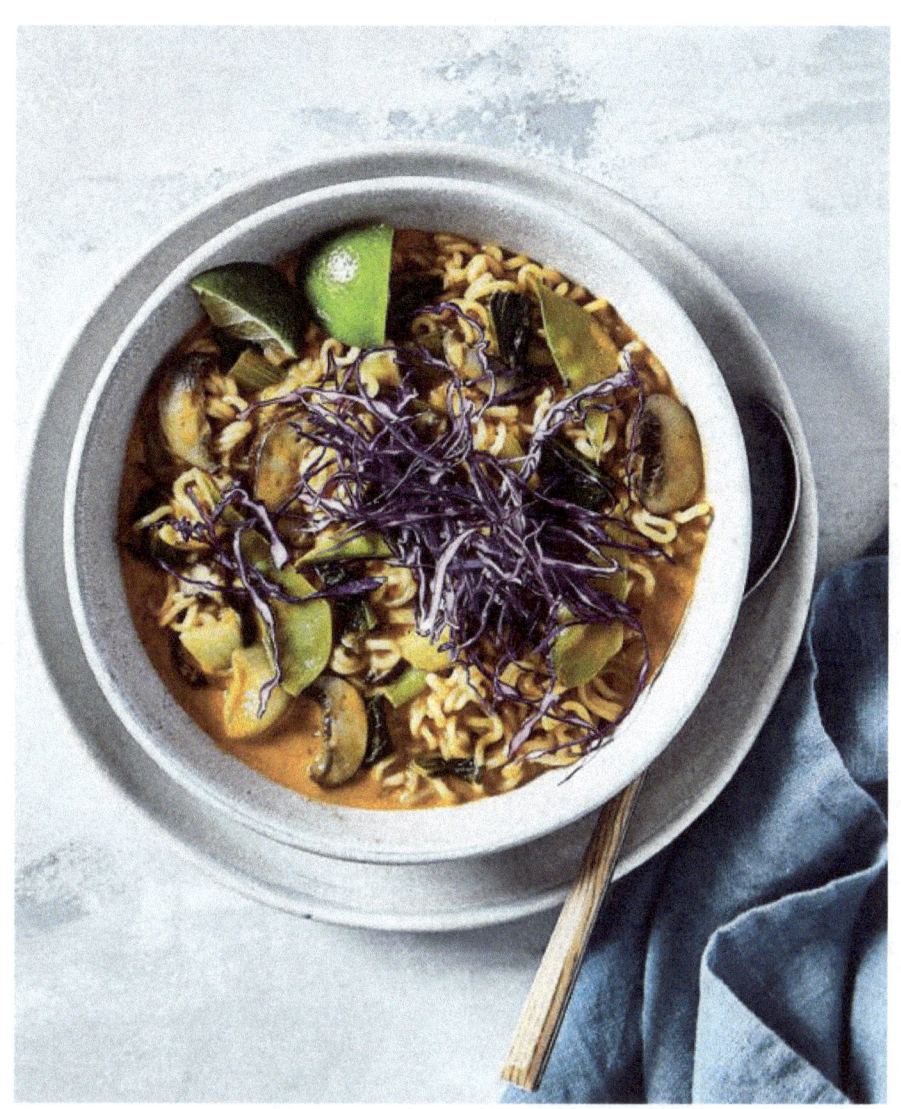

Coconut Curry Ramen

PREP TIME: 10 minutes

COOK TIME: 15 minutes

OIL-FREE, ONE POT, SOY-FREE

SERVES 4

Instant ramen noodles get a grown-up makeover in this soupy noodle dish, though they can be swapped out for shirataki noodles or spiralized zucchini noodles for a healthier take. The heat from Thai red curry paste is balanced perfectly with creamy coconut milk and the bright acidity of lime. I top this ramen with red cabbage because the color is such a great contrast with the orange-hued soup, and it adds great texture, but if you don't like cabbage, chunks of avocado would be just as delicious.

2 to 3 tablespoons Thai red curry paste

2 teaspoons grated ginger

1 teaspoon minced garlic

2 baby bok choy heads, coarsely chopped

6 cremini mushrooms, stems removed and caps sliced

1 (13.5-ounce) can full-fat coconut milk

1 cup snow peas, halved

⅔ cup low-sodium vegetable broth

4 (3-ounce) packages instant ramen noodles (seasoning packets discarded)

3 cups shredded red cabbage

1 lime, quartered, for garnish

1. In a large pot, heat the curry paste, ginger, and garlic over medium heat for 2 minutes, until fragrant. Add the bok choy, mushrooms, coconut milk, snow peas, and vegetable broth and bring to a simmer. Cook for 10 minutes.

2. Add the ramen noodles to the pot and cook for another 3 minutes,

tossing the ramen until coated.

3. Divide into bowls, top with the shredded cabbage, and serve with lime wedges.

PER SERVING: Calories: 596; Fat: 32g; Protein: 13g; Carbohydrates: 68g; Fiber: 7g

Sweet Potato and Spinach Curry

PREP TIME: 10 minutes

COOK TIME: 20 minutes

GLUTEN-FREE, ONE POT, SOY-FREE

SERVES 4

I love how hearty this curry is, and how rich and bright the flavors are. It's my go-to winter dish when I'm craving something that will warm me to my core. The trick to making this in under 30 minutes is to dice the sweet potatoes very small so that they will cook faster. If you have a can or bag of peas and carrots, use them here for extra color and flavor.

1 tablespoon grapeseed or extra-virgin olive oil

½ medium onion, diced

1 cup canned diced tomatoes, drained

3 tablespoons Everyday Curry Paste or store-bought mild curry paste

2 medium sweet potatoes, peeled and cut into ½-inch cubes

1 (15-ounce) can chickpeas, drained and rinsed

1 (13.5-ounce) can full-fat coconut milk

½ cup low-sodium vegetable

broth 8 ounces baby spinach

Juice of 1 lime

1. In a Dutch oven or large sauté pan with a tight-fitting lid, heat the oil on medium-high heat. Add the onion and cook for 4 minutes, until just translucent. Add the tomatoes and curry paste and stir until just warmed through and fragrant, about 30 seconds.

2. Add the sweet potatoes, chickpeas, coconut milk, and vegetable broth. Bring to a simmer, cover, and cook for about 15 minutes, until the potatoes are tender.

3. Remove from the heat, add the spinach and lime juice, and stir until the spinach is wilted. Serve.

PER SERVING: Calories: 406; Fat: 25g; Protein: 10g; Carbohydrates: 43g; Fiber: 11g

Butter Chicken Tofu

PREP TIME: 10 minutes

COOK TIME: 20 minutes

GLUTEN-FREE, ONE POT

SERVES 5

Butter chicken is a classic Indian dish, made from a rich cream-and-tomato-based curry sauce. I use full-fat coconut milk to give this version a rich and creamy texture, and a good amount of cayenne to give it some heat. Feel free to adjust the heat to your taste or swap it for paprika to add flavor without adding spice. I love serving this dish with basmati rice, quinoa, or vegan naan.

2 tablespoons grapeseed or extra-virgin olive oil, divided

2 (14-ounce) blocks extra-firm tofu, cut into ½-inch cubes

3 tablespoons cornstarch

1 medium onion, diced

1 tablespoon grated ginger

1 teaspoon minced garlic

1 (13.5-ounce) full-fat coconut milk

¼ cup plus 2 tablespoons tomato

paste 1 tablespoon ground cumin

1 teaspoon mild curry

powder ½ teaspoon salt

¼ to ½ teaspoon ground cayenne pepper

1. In a large sauté pan or skillet, heat 1 tablespoon of oil on medium-high heat. In a large resealable bag, combine the tofu and cornstarch and shake well until coated. Add the tofu to the hot pan and cook until crispy on all sides, about 6 minutes. Transfer the tofu to a plate and return the pan to the heat.

2. Add the remaining 1 tablespoon of oil to the pan, along with the

onion. Cook the onion for 3 to 4 minutes, or until just translucent. Add the ginger and garlic and cook, stirring constantly, for 30 seconds, until fragrant.

3. Add the coconut milk, tomato paste, cumin, curry powder, salt, and cayenne. Stir to combine and simmer for 10 minutes, until the sauce is bubbling and thickens slightly. Return the tofu to the pan and toss to coat. Serve with rice or vegan naan.

PER SERVING: Calories: 396; Fat: 28g; Protein: 19g; Carbohydrates: 21g; Fiber: 4g

Yellow Curried Chickpeas with Kale

PREP TIME: 10 minutes

COOK TIME: 20 minutes

GLUTEN-FREE, ONE POT, SOY-FREE

SERVES 6

I have a favorite lentil curry stew recipe that I keep on repeat all winter long. It's warm and thick and comforting and I could pretty much live on it. But it requires cooking dry lentils, which takes much longer than 30 minutes on a stovetop. So I adapted that recipe into a quick and easy curried chickpea recipe using canned chickpeas. It has all the flavor of the lentil version, but with less work. Serve with quinoa or rice, or on its own.

1 tablespoon grapeseed or extra-virgin olive oil

½ medium onion, diced

1 large carrot, diced

2 tablespoons mild curry powder

1½ teaspoons minced garlic

1 teaspoon grated ginger

½ teaspoon paprika

½ teaspoon smoked paprika

¼ to ½ teaspoon ground cayenne

pepper 4 cups chopped kale

2 (15-ounce) cans chickpeas, drained and rinsed

1 (13.5-ounce) can full-fat coconut milk

½ cup low-sodium vegetable

broth Juice of 1 lime

1. In a large pot, heat the oil on medium-high heat. Add the onion and carrot and cook for about 5 minutes, until the onion is translucent. Add the curry powder, garlic, ginger, paprika, smoked paprika, and cayenne and cook, stirring constantly, for 30 seconds until the carrot and onion are coated and the spices are fragrant.

2. Add the kale, chickpeas, coconut milk, and vegetable broth. Bring to a boil, then reduce the heat to medium and simmer for 15 minutes. Add the lime juice and serve.

PER SERVING: Calories: 277; Fat: 16g; Protein: 8g; Carbohydrates: 28g; Fiber: 9g

Stir-Fried Teriyaki Udon Bowl

PREP TIME: 10 minutes

COOK TIME: 15 minutes

NUT-FREE

SERVES 3

I grew up hanging out at the mall and eating mall food. One of my favorites was the udon teriyaki from the quick-serve Japanese restaurant in the food court. Crisp, crunchy vegetables, slurpy noodles, and protein stir-fried with a delicious teriyaki sauce. This recipe is an homage to that dish, but without the 20-minute struggle to find a parking spot!

½ cup cold water

2 tablespoons low-sodium soy sauce

1 tablespoon brown sugar

2 teaspoons cornstarch

1 teaspoon maple syrup

¼ teaspoon grated ginger

¼ teaspoon garlic powder

2 (7-ounce) packages udon noodles

1 tablespoon grapeseed or extra-virgin olive oil

1 (14-ounce) block tofu, drained, pressed, and cut into ½-inch cubes

1 (8-ounce) bag shredded coleslaw mix

1 cup snow peas, halved

1. In a small bowl, whisk the water, soy sauce, brown sugar, cornstarch, maple syrup, ginger, and garlic powder until smooth. Set aside.

2. Bring a large pot of water to a boil and cook the udon noodles according to package directions.

3. While the noodles are cooking, in a large sauté pan or skillet, heat the oil on medium-high heat. Add the tofu and cook until crispy on all sides, about 7 minutes. Add the coleslaw mix and snow peas and cook

for another 3 to 4 minutes, tossing frequently, until the vegetables are soft.

4. Drain the noodles, add the noodles and the soy sauce mixture to the pan, and toss to combine. Cook for 2 minutes, or until the sauce thickens and coats the noodles and tofu. Serve.

PER SERVING: Calories: 687; Fat: 15g; Protein: 36g; Carbohydrates: 105g; Fiber: 11g

7

Soups, Stews, and Chilis

Vegetable Pho
Spicy Corn Chowder
Tortilla Soup
Broccoli Cheddar Soup
Spicy Peanut Satay Ramen
Tempeh Barbecue Chili
Lemony Split Pea Soup
Sweet Potato Coconut Curry Stew
Creamy Vegetable Soup
Chickpea and Potato Stew
Tomato Basil Gnocchi Soup
Chili Rice and Beans
Tofu Shakshuka
Creamy Lasagna Soup
Pasta e Fagioli

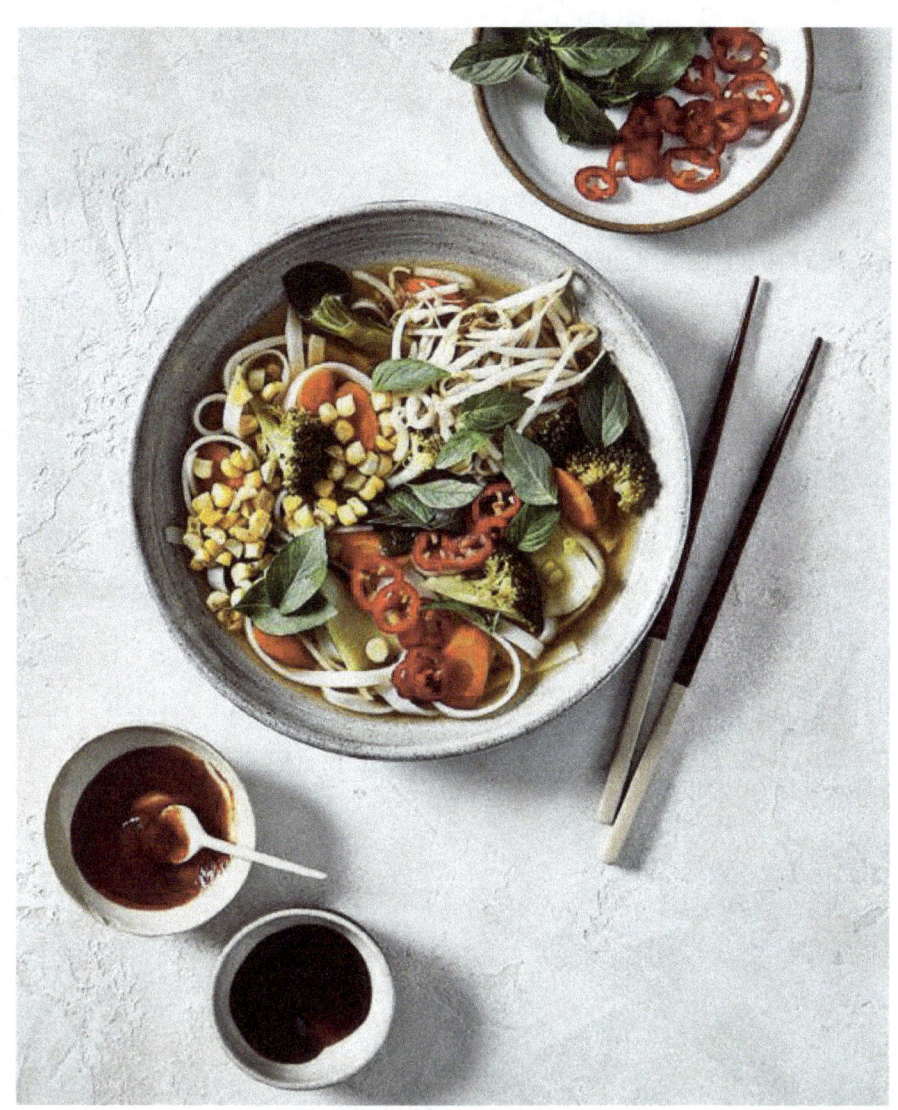

Vegetable Pho

PREP TIME: 10 minutes

COOK TIME: 20 minutes

GLUTEN-FREE, NUT-FREE, OIL-FREE

SERVES 6

Vietnamese pho is a classic noodle soup full of aromatic flavors like ginger, cinnamon, star anise, garlic, and clove. This recipe simmers whole spices in broth to make an authentic soup, but if you're in a hurry, or you can't find those spices near you, many supermarkets sell vegetarian pho broth in the soup aisle. Just bring it to a slight boil, add the veggies, and in less than 10 minutes you've got dinner.

For the broth

8 cups low-sodium vegetable broth

3 cups water

1 large onion, quartered

1 cinnamon stick

3 whole star anise

3 whole cloves

2-inch piece fresh ginger, peeled

2 garlic cloves, halved

2 tablespoons tamari

8 ounces wide rice noodles

3 baby bok choy heads, separated into individual leaves

2 cups broccoli florets

2 carrots, thinly sliced

2 scallions, both green and white parts, chopped

For serving

1 (15-ounce) can corn, drained

1 cup bean sprouts

1 jalapeño or Thai chile pepper, sliced into rings
1 bunch fresh basil leaves (Thai or Italian)
Sriracha
Hoisin sauce

1. In a large pot, combine the broth, water, onion, cinnamon, anise, cloves, ginger, garlic, and tamari and bring almost to a boil. Reduce the heat slightly and simmer, covered, for 20 minutes.

2. While the soup is cooking, bring a medium pot of water to a boil and cook the rice noodles according to package directions. Drain.

3. During the last 5 minutes of the broth's cooking time, add the bok choy, broccoli, carrots, and scallions.

4. To serve: Ladle the soup into bowls and add the noodles. Top with corn, bean sprouts, jalapeño, and basil leaves. Season with sriracha and hoisin sauce to taste.

PER SERVING: Calories: 230; Fat: 1g; Protein: 7g; Carbohydrates: 49g; Fiber: 4g

Spicy Corn Chowder

PREP TIME: 5 minutes

COOK TIME: 20 minutes

EASY PREP, GLUTEN-FREE, OIL-FREE, ONE POT, SOY-FREE

SERVES 8

This is my go-to winter soup. I live in a climate where winter is really cold, and eating a hot bowl of this soup is like being warmed up from the inside. It's full of rich, spicy, smoky flavors from the chipotle powder. I like to use chipotle because it adds depth as well as heat. It is strong, though, so don't use more than the recipe calls for or your soup will smell like a campfire.

2 medium yellow potatoes, peeled and cut into 1-inch cubes

2 cups low-sodium vegetable broth

1 (13.5-ounce) can full-fat coconut milk

1 (16-ounce) bag frozen corn

2 tablespoons nutritional yeast

1 teaspoon chipotle powder

1 teaspoon canned diced green chiles, drained

½ teaspoon ground mustard

½ teaspoon paprika

1. In a large pot, combine the potatoes, vegetable broth, coconut milk, corn, nutritional yeast, chipotle powder, green chiles, mustard, and paprika and stir to combine. Bring to a soft boil and reduce the heat to medium-low. Cover and simmer for 25 minutes, until the potatoes are tender.

2. Remove the soup from the heat and partially blend with a stick blender, or transfer to a stand blender in small batches and partially blend, leaving some of the soup chunky. Return to the pot and serve.

PER SERVING: Calories: 176; Fat: 9g; Protein: 5g; Carbohydrates: 24g; Fiber: 3g

Tortilla Soup

PREP TIME: 10 minutes

COOK TIME: 20 minutes

GLUTEN-FREE, NUT-FREE, SOY-FREE

SERVES 4

Tortilla soup is a traditional Mexican dish made with fried tortilla pieces and served in a rich, spicy tomato-based broth. For this version, we're baking the tortilla strips to make them healthier but still full of great spice and flavor. You can dial up or down the amount of heat in this dish and switch out the beans and vegetables to use whatever you have on hand.

6 (6-inch) corn or flour tortillas, cut into strips

2 tablespoons grapeseed or extra-virgin olive oil, divided

¾ teaspoon salt, divided

1 medium onion, diced

1 jalapeño pepper, sliced into rings or 2 tablespoons canned chopped jalapeños 1 teaspoon minced garlic

1 teaspoon ground cumin

1 teaspoon chili powder

½ teaspoon freshly ground black pepper ¼ to ½ teaspoon ground cayenne pepper 4 cups low-sodium vegetable broth

1 (28-ounce) can crushed tomatoes

2 cups frozen mixed vegetables (corn, carrots, peas, green beans) 1 (15-ounce) can black beans, drained and rinsed

Optional toppings: diced avocado, shredded pepper Jack–style vegan cheese, vegan sour cream, chopped fresh cilantro

1. Preheat the oven to 475°F and line a rimmed baking sheet with parchment paper.

2. Stack the tortillas and cut in half, then cut into strips about ½ inch wide. Toss with 1 tablespoon of oil and spread in a single layer on the

prepared sheet. Bake for 6 to 7 minutes, or until lightly golden. Remove from the pan, sprinkle with ¼ teaspoon of salt, and set aside.

3. In a large pot, heat the remaining 1 tablespoon of oil on medium-high heat. Add the onion and cook for 3 to 4 minutes, or until just translucent. Add the jalapeño, garlic, cumin, chili powder, black pepper, remaining ½ teaspoon of salt, and cayenne pepper and cook for 30 seconds, until fragrant.

4. Pour in the broth and tomatoes. Bring to a boil, then reduce the heat to medium and simmer for 5 minutes.

5. Add the frozen vegetables and black beans and cook for another 3 to 4 minutes, or until the vegetables are warmed through. Serve in bowls topped with tortilla strips and your choice of toppings.

PER SERVING: Calories: 363; Fat: 9g; Protein: 13g; Carbohydrates: 59g; Fiber: 16g

Broccoli Cheddar Soup

PREP TIME: 10 minutes

COOK TIME: 20 minutes

GLUTEN-FREE, ONE POT, SOY-FREE

SERVES 6

This is my mother-in-law's favorite soup. She's not plant-based, but she swears this soup is just as good as a dairy-laden version, only she feels much better after she eats this one. I've added extra protein to this soup by using white beans as a thickener instead of flour.

1 tablespoon grapeseed or extra-virgin olive oil

1 medium onion, diced

3 cups low-sodium vegetable broth

1 (12-ounce) bag broccoli florets

1 cup canned cannellini or white kidney beans, drained and rinsed

¾ cup canned full-fat coconut milk

¾ cup shredded Cheddar-style vegan

cheese 2 tablespoons nutritional yeast

1 teaspoon ground

mustard Salt

Freshly ground black pepper

1. In a large pot, heat the oil on medium-high heat. Add the onion and cook for about 4 minutes, until just translucent and soft. Add the vegetable broth, broccoli, and beans. Bring to a boil, then reduce the heat to medium and simmer for 10 minutes.

2. Remove from the heat and puree completely with a stick blender (or in a stand blender, working in small batches).

3. Return the pot to the stovetop on medium heat. Add the coconut milk, cheese, nutritional yeast, and mustard and simmer, stirring frequently, for about 7 minutes, until warmed through and the cheese

has melted. Season with salt and pepper to taste.

VARY IT: Turn this soup into a loaded-baked-potato soup by crumbling tofu "bacon" on top and adding a dollop of vegan sour cream and some diced scallions or chives. To make the tofu bacon, in a small bowl, whisk together 2 tablespoons soy sauce, 1 tablespoon maple syrup, 1 tablespoon apple cider vinegar, and 2 to 3 drops liquid smoke. In a large sauté pan or skillet, heat 1 tablespoon oil on medium-high heat and add 14 ounces extra-firm tofu, cut into strips. Cook for 5 minutes per side, or until golden, then pour in the sauce and continue cooking until the strips are sticky and caramelized, about 3 minutes. Dice them up and serve in the soup.

PER SERVING: Calories: 185; Fat: 11g; Protein: 6g; Carbohydrates: 18g; Fiber: 4g

Spicy Peanut Satay Ramen

PREP TIME: 5 minutes

COOK TIME: 15 minutes

EASY PREP, ONE POT

SERVES 4

When I'm in a hurry but need something filling, warm, and delicious for dinner, this is my go-to. It's got the perfect balance of hot, sweet, spicy, and savory and is a perfect canvas for using up any veggies I have lying around, or for eating on its own. This recipe will yield a very soupy ramen.

1 teaspoon sesame oil

3 scallions, both white and green parts, chopped and divided

2 teaspoons minced garlic

1 teaspoon grated ginger

1 teaspoon Thai red curry paste

4 cups low-sodium vegetable broth

1 (13.5-ounce) can full-fat coconut milk

½ cup creamy peanut butter

2 tablespoons tamari or dark soy sauce

2 tablespoons maple syrup

Juice of 2 limes, plus 1 lime, quartered, for garnish

3 (3-ounce) packages ramen noodles (seasoning packets discarded)

½ cup canned sliced or shredded bamboo

shoots ¼ cup crushed peanuts

1. In a large pot, heat the oil on medium-high heat. Add the white parts of the scallions, garlic, ginger, and curry paste and cook for 1 to 2 minutes, stirring constantly, until fragrant. Add the vegetable broth, coconut milk, peanut butter, tamari, maple syrup, and lime juice and stir well to combine. Reduce the heat to low and simmer for 10 minutes.

2. Add the ramen noodles and bamboo shoots to the pot and cook for 2 to 3 minutes, or until done. Serve topped with the crushed peanuts and scallion greens.

PER SERVING: Calories: 769; Fat: 50g; Protein: 19g; Carbohydrates: 65g; Fiber: 7g

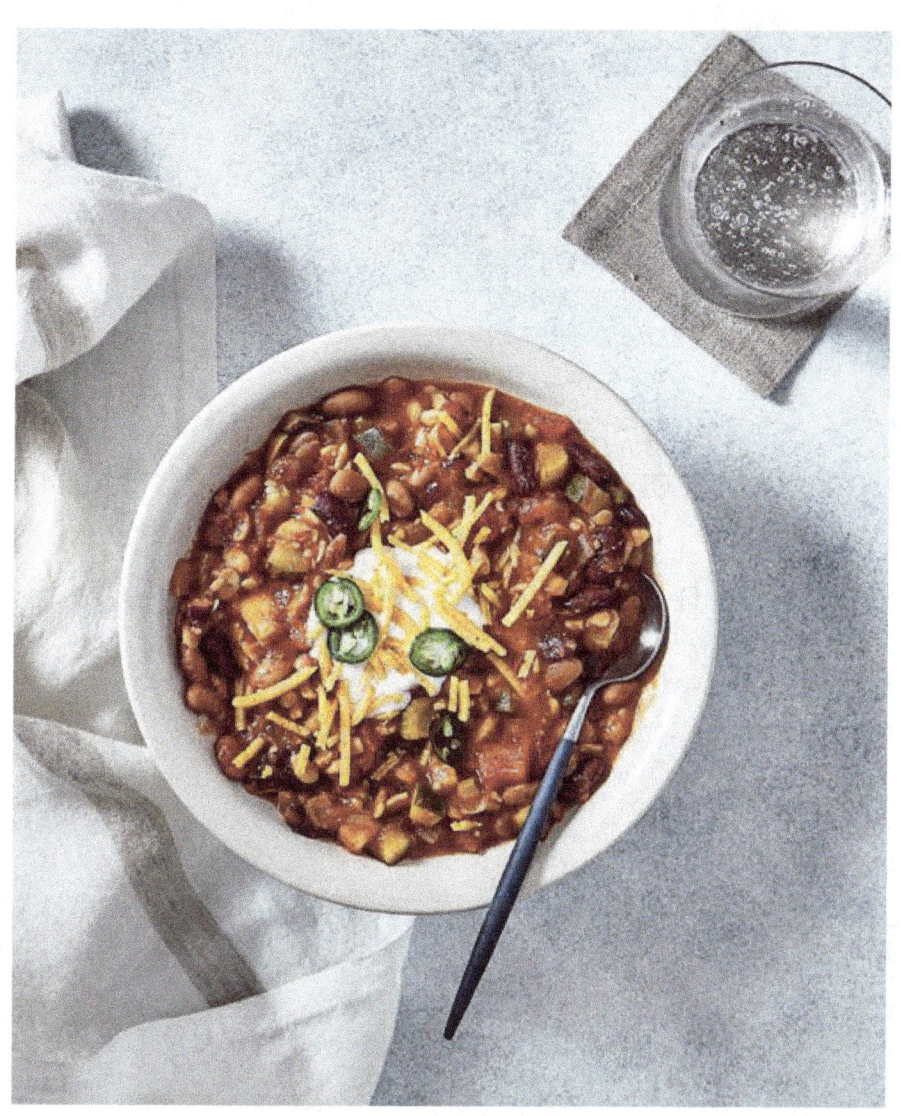

Tempeh Barbecue Chili

PREP TIME: 10 minutes

COOK TIME: 20 minutes

GLUTEN-FREE, NUT-FREE, ONE POT

SERVES 4

This protein- and fiber-packed chili is just hot enough to wake up your taste buds. I like to sneak extra vegetables into my chili—especially when I'm making it for my kids, who eat it as a taco filing and can't *see* the vegetables.

2 tablespoons grapeseed or extra-virgin olive oil

1 (7-ounce) package tempeh, crumbled or grated

1 medium onion, diced

1 green zucchini, diced

1 yellow summer squash, diced

2 celery stalks, diced

1 teaspoon minced garlic

1 (15-ounce) can pinto beans, drained and rinsed

1 (15-ounce) can kidney beans, drained and rinsed

¾ cup water

¾ cup tomato sauce

½ cup canned diced tomatoes, drained and

rinsed ¼ cup vegan barbecue sauce

1 tablespoon maple syrup

1 tablespoon chili powder

¼ teaspoon ground cayenne pepper or red pepper flakes

1. In a large pot, heat the oil on medium-high heat. Add the tempeh, onion, zucchini, summer squash, celery, and garlic. Cook until the tempeh is browned and the onion is translucent, about 5 minutes.

2. Add the pinto and kidney beans, water, tomato sauce, tomatoes, barbecue sauce, maple syrup, chili powder, and cayenne. Bring to a boil, then reduce the heat to medium and simmer for 15 minutes,

until the flavors meld.

3. To serve: Divide the chili into bowls and top each bowl with your favorite chili toppings. See the tip below for some recommendations.

INGREDIENT TIP: Experiment with different toppings to find your favorite combination. In my house, we love vegan sour cream, shredded Cheddar-style vegan cheese, and sliced jalapeño peppers (either fresh or pickled).

PER SERVING: Calories: 483; Fat: 19g; Protein: 25g; Carbohydrates: 60g; Fiber: 15g

Lemony Split Pea Soup

PREP TIME: 5 minutes

COOK TIME: 25 minutes

EASY PREP, GLUTEN-FREE, OIL-FREE, ONE POT, SOY-FREE

SERVES 8

Growing up in a climate where winter is real—and long—stick-to-your-ribs soups are a necessity. Years ago, I wrote a "weekend" version of this soup that simmers low and slow, with chunks of vegetables and aromatics, but I needed a version that worked on busy days too. Because split peas need a good 20 to 25 minutes in the pot to soften, I've skipped the extra prep and opted for canned vegetables and spices to flavor this soup.

6 cups low-sodium vegetable broth
1½ cups yellow split peas, rinsed
1 (8.5-ounce) can sliced carrots, drained
1 cup canned corn, drained
2 teaspoons ground cumin
1 teaspoon onion powder
1 teaspoon garlic powder
1 teaspoon mild curry powder
⅛ teaspoon ground turmeric
⅛ teaspoon ground cayenne
pepper ¼ cup canned full-fat
coconut milk Juice and grated
zest of 1 lemon Salt
Freshly ground black pepper

1. In a large pot, combine the vegetable broth, split peas, carrots, corn, cumin, onion powder, garlic powder, curry powder, turmeric, and cayenne. Stir well. Bring to a boil, reduce the heat to medium, and

simmer for 25 minutes, until the split peas are tender.

2. Remove from the heat and stir in the coconut milk and lemon juice and zest. Season with salt and black pepper and serve.

TECHNIQUE TIP: To give this soup a creamier texture, use a stick blender to puree the soup (adding a little extra coconut milk to loosen if needed), or working in small batches, blend it in a stand blender.

PER SERVING: Calories: 179; Fat: 3g; Protein: 9g; Carbohydrates: 31g; Fiber: 10g

Sweet Potato Coconut Curry Stew

PREP TIME: 10 minutes

COOK TIME: 20 minutes

GLUTEN-FREE, ONE POT, SOY-FREE

SERVES 4

Sweet potatoes are an incredibly delicious and colorful way to get extra fiber and vitamins into your diet and are a nice change from traditional white potatoes. Cutting sweet potatoes into small chunks helps them cook faster, making this stew an easy and healthy 30-minute meal. If your grocery store has peeled and chopped fresh sweet potatoes, use those and save yourself some prep time.

1 tablespoon grapeseed or extra-virgin olive oil

2 medium sweet potatoes, peeled and cut into 1-inch cubes

1 medium onion, diced

1 large carrot, diced

1 tablespoon mild curry powder

½ teaspoon ground cumin

½ teaspoon salt

½ teaspoon freshly ground black pepper ¼ teaspoon ground cinnamon

3½ cups low-sodium vegetable broth

½ cup full-fat coconut milk

1 (15-ounce) can lentils, drained and rinsed

1. In a large pot, heat the oil on medium-high heat. Add the sweet potatoes, onion, carrot, curry powder, cumin, salt, pepper, and cinnamon and cook for 2 minutes, until the spices are fragrant.

2. Add the vegetable broth and coconut milk and bring to a boil. Reduce the heat to medium and simmer for 15 minutes. Add the lentils and cook for another 5 minutes, until the flavors meld.

PER SERVING: Calories: 273; Fat: 10g; Protein: 11g; Carbohydrates: 39g; Fiber: 9g

Creamy Vegetable Soup

PREP TIME: 10 minutes

COOK TIME: 15 minutes

GLUTEN-FREE, NUT-FREE, ONE POT

SERVES 6

Vegetable soup is a great dish to make when you're looking to use up fresh or frozen vegetables. This version has a creamy, thick texture through the addition of potatoes and soy milk. To shorten prep and cook time, I use frozen diced potatoes.

1 tablespoon grapeseed or extra-virgin olive oil

2 large carrots, diced

2 celery stalks, diced

1 medium onion, diced

1 teaspoon dried dill

3 cups low-sodium vegetable broth

1 vegan chicken bouillon cube

3 cups frozen diced potatoes

2 cups frozen peas

2 cups frozen corn

2 cups unsweetened soy milk

1. In a large pot, heat the oil on medium-high heat. Add the carrots, celery, onion, and dill and cook for about 5 minutes, until the onion is just translucent and the celery and carrots start to soften. Add the vegetable broth and bouillon and bring to a boil.

2. Reduce the heat to medium, add the potatoes, and simmer for 10 minutes. Add the peas, corn, and soy milk and stir to combine.

3. Remove from the heat and partially puree, using a stick blender (or blend half of the soup in a stand blender in small batches and return to the pot). Serve.

INGREDIENT TIP: If you can't find vegan chicken-flavored bouillon, substitute with vegetable bouillon. It gives the soup that "simmered for hours" flavor in just a few minutes.

PER SERVING: Calories: 227; Fat: g; Protein: 9g; Carbohydrates: 40g; Fiber: 6g

Chickpea and Potato Stew

PREP TIME: 5 minutes

COOK TIME: 15 minutes

EASY PREP, GLUTEN-FREE, ONE POT, SOY-FREE

SERVES 5

No matter how busy your day is, you can have this comforting dish on the table in under 20 minutes. A short ingredient list and quick-cooking hacks like using frozen diced or hash brown potatoes are the keys to keeping this dish no-fuss. This stew is great on its own, or in a sandwich wrap. If you've got some frozen or canned peas and carrots on hand, add them at the end to brighten the dish even more.

1 tablespoon grapeseed or extra-virgin olive oil

4 cups frozen diced or hash brown potatoes

1 medium onion, diced

2 (15-ounce) cans chickpeas, drained and rinsed

2 tablespoons Everyday Curry Paste or store-bought mild curry paste

2 (13.5-ounce) cans full-fat coconut milk

1. In a large pot, heat the oil on medium-high heat. Add the potatoes and onion and cook for about 5 minutes, until the onion is translucent and the potatoes start to soften. Add the chickpeas and curry paste and stir to combine.

2. Pour in the coconut milk, reduce the heat to medium-low, and simmer for 10 minutes, or until the sauce thickens slightly. Serve.

VARY IT: To give this dish a Tex-Mex twist, divide the filling among 10-inch whole-wheat tortillas and roll them up into burritos. Place in a lightly greased baking dish and cover with more curry sauce and shredded cheese, such as a vegan Monterey Jack. Bake for 10 minutes and you've got curried chickpea potato enchiladas.

PER SERVING: Calories: 588; Fat: 34g; Protein: 13g; Carbohydrates: 64g; Fiber: 11g

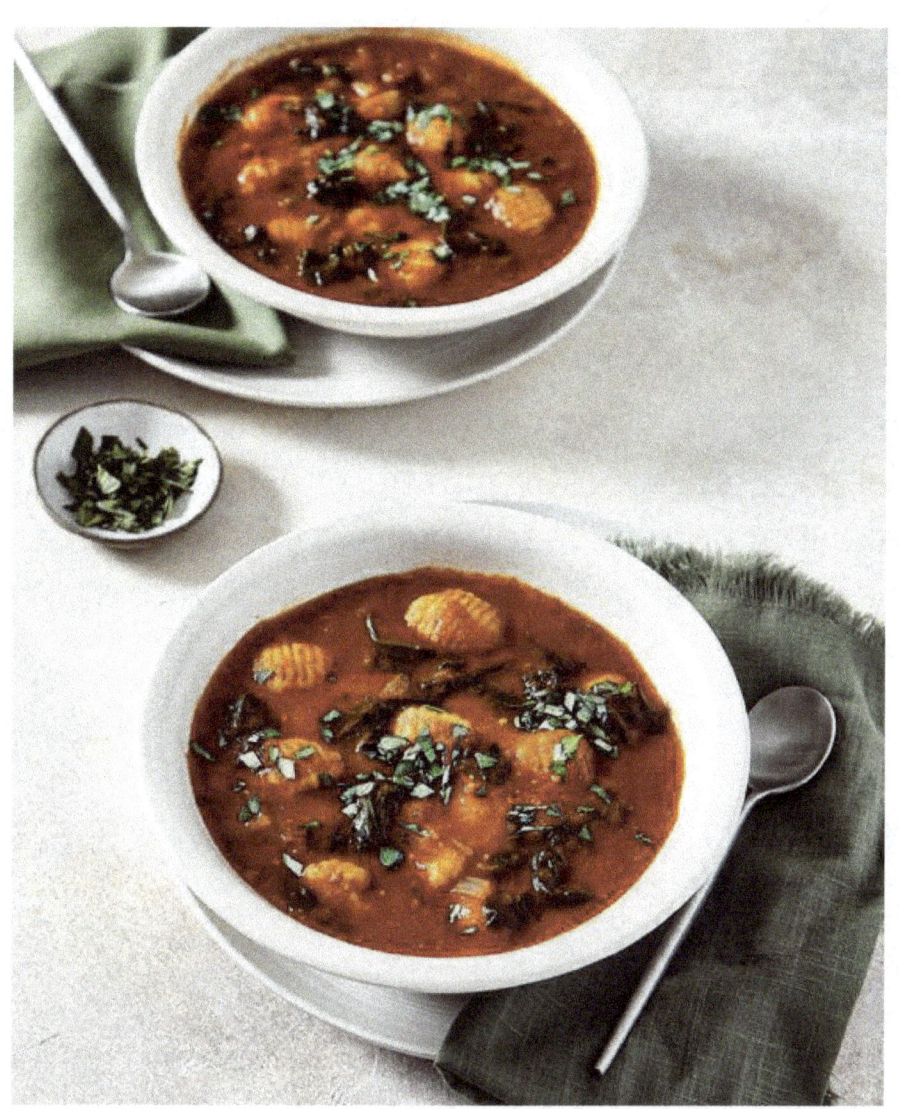

Tomato Basil Gnocchi Soup

PREP TIME: 5 minutes

COOK TIME: 10 minutes

EASY PREP, NUT-FREE, ONE POT, SOY-FREE, SUPERFAST

SERVES 4

I was never a huge fan of gnocchi until I tried it in this soup. I ate this dish in a restaurant years ago and knew I had to find a way to make it at home. Ready-made tomato sauce and fresh gnocchi make this the perfect quick lunch or dinner. And it's a definite step up from regular tomato soup.

1 tablespoon grapeseed or extra-virgin olive oil
4 cups fresh baby spinach
1 medium onion, diced
1½ teaspoons minced garlic
1 teaspoon freshly squeezed lemon juice
3 cups tomato-basil pasta sauce
3 cups low-sodium vegetable broth
24 ounces fresh vegan gnocchi
2 tablespoons nutritional yeast
Salt
Freshly ground black pepper
2 tablespoons chopped fresh basil, for garnish

1. In a large pot, heat the oil on medium-high heat. Add the baby spinach, onion, garlic, and lemon juice and cook for 5 minutes, or until the onion is translucent and the spinach is soft.

2. Add the pasta sauce and vegetable broth and bring to a simmer. Add the gnocchi and cook for 3 minutes, or until tender.

3. Remove from the heat, stir in the nutritional yeast, and season with salt and pepper. Garnish with fresh basil and serve.

VARY IT: For some extra richness (and if you don't need the recipe to be nut-free or soy-free), stir a couple tablespoons of coconut or soy cream into each bowl before serving.

PER SERVING: Calories: 375; Fat: 16g; Protein: 11g; Carbohydrates: 48g; Fiber: 7g

Chili Rice and Beans

PREP TIME: 10 minutes

COOK TIME: 15 minutes

GLUTEN-FREE, NUT-FREE, SOY-FREE

SERVES 4

This recipe is great as a meal on its own or as a fancy side dish. When I need something satisfying on the table in under 30 minutes, I serve this as a main course. But if I have a little extra time, it's a fantastic filling for stuffed peppers or even for enchiladas (just swap the paprika for chili powder to give this dish a Tex-Mex flavor profile).

2 cups low-sodium vegetable broth

1 cup basmati or long-grain white rice, rinsed

3 tablespoons tomato sauce

1½ tablespoons Italian seasoning

½ teaspoon paprika

½ teaspoon salt

½ teaspoon freshly ground black pepper

1 tablespoon grapeseed or extra-virgin olive oil

1 medium onion, diced

1 green bell pepper, diced

1 red bell pepper, diced

1 large zucchini, diced

1 (15-ounce) can black beans, drained and rinsed

1. In a medium pot, combine the vegetable broth, rice, tomato sauce, Italian seasoning, paprika, salt, and pepper. Stir well. Bring to a boil, then reduce the heat to low, cover, and cook for 15 minutes, or until the rice is tender and the liquid is absorbed. Set aside when done.

2. While the rice is cooking, in a large sauté pan or skillet, heat the oil on medium-high heat. Add the onion, bell peppers, and zucchini and

cook for 6 to 8 minutes, until the onion is soft and the peppers and zucchini are fork-tender.

3. Add the cooked rice and drained beans to the pan with the vegetables and toss to combine. Stir for about 1 minute, until the beans are warmed through.

STRETCH IT: Use the leftovers from this dish as a burrito or bowl filling with shredded vegan cheese and diced avocado.

PER SERVING: Calories: 348; Fat: 5g; Protein: 12g; Carbohydrates: 67g; Fiber: 11g

Tofu Shakshuka

PREP TIME: 10 minutes

COOK TIME: 20 minutes

GLUTEN-FREE, NUT-FREE, OIL-FREE

SERVES 4

This recipe takes a bit of work, but the result is worth it. Shakshuka is a traditional Mediterranean dish, combining tomatoes, onion, garlic, and spices to make a chunky sauce in which eggs are poached. I recreate that flavorful, spicy sauce and use a vegan egg yolk sauce to replicate the poached egg. Bookmark this yolk recipe—you'll want to use it everywhere.

1 cup cold water

2 tablespoons unsweetened soy milk

1 tablespoon cornstarch

2 teaspoons nutritional yeast

½ teaspoon black salt (optional)

¼ teaspoon ground turmeric

1 (14-ounce) block firm tofu, drained and pressed

1 (28-ounce) can Italian seasoned diced tomatoes

2 teaspoons minced garlic

1 teaspoon ground cumin

½ teaspoon paprika

½ teaspoon salt

½ teaspoon freshly ground black pepper

1. In a small saucepan, whisk together the water, soy milk, cornstarch, nutritional yeast, black salt (if using), and turmeric. Heat over medium-high heat and cook for 5 minutes, or until the sauce thickens. This is the vegan "yolk." Set aside.

2. Cut the tofu block in half lengthwise and then into rounds using a small cookie cutter. Set aside.

3. In a large sauté pan or skillet, combine the tomatoes and their juices, garlic, cumin, paprika, salt, and pepper. Heat over medium heat and let simmer for 5 minutes, until it's just warmed through and starting to bubble.

4. Dip the tofu rounds in the vegan yolk mixture, then add them to the tomato mixture, making little wells in the sauce to "cradle" the tofu. Simmer for 10 minutes, until warmed through.

INGREDIENT TIP: Also known as Himalayan black salt, or kala namak, black salt is actually a pinkish-gray color and has its origins in South Asia. It has a naturally sulfurous smell similar to that of hard-boiled eggs. Plant-based eaters often use kala namak mixed with nutritional yeast and turmeric to give tofu dishes a distinctly "eggy" flavor.

PER SERVING: Calories: 170; Fat: 5g; Protein: 13g; Carbohydrates: 18g; Fiber: 5g

Creamy Lasagna Soup

PREP TIME: 10 minutes

COOK TIME: 15 minutes

SOY-FREE

SERVES 6

I had no idea until recently that lasagna soup was a thing. Apparently, it's a big thing. But every version I've seen was tomato-based, and since I have non-tomato-sauce-loving kids, I wanted to create a version for them that had a cream base, much like alfredo sauce. The soup comes together while the noodles cook, making this an easy dish to prepare in under 30 minutes.

1 (16-ounce) box lasagna noodles

1 tablespoon grapeseed or extra-virgin olive oil

6 ounces cremini mushrooms, stems removed and caps sliced

1 medium onion, diced

1 teaspoon minced garlic

3 cups low-sodium vegetable broth

1 (13.5-ounce) can full-fat coconut milk

2 tablespoons nutritional yeast

1 vegan chicken bouillon cube

1 cup shredded mozzarella-style vegan cheese

½ teaspoon freshly ground black pepper

2 tablespoons chopped fresh flat-leaf parsley, for garnish (optional)

1. Bring a large pot of water to a boil and cook the lasagna noodles according to package directions. Drain and rinse under cold water and set aside.

2. While the noodles are cooking, in a large pot, heat the oil on medium-high heat. Add the mushrooms, onion, and garlic and cook for about 6 minutes, stirring frequently, until the onion is translucent,

and the mushrooms are softened.

3. Add the vegetable broth, coconut milk, nutritional yeast, and bouillon cube and bring to a light boil over medium-high heat, then reduce the heat to medium-low. Stir in the mozzarella and pepper and simmer for about 5 minutes, until the cheese melts.

4. Tear or cut the cooked lasagna noodles into strips and add to the soup. Garnish with parsley (if using) and serve.

PER SERVING: Calories: 498; Fat: 19g; Protein: 14g; Carbohydrates: 70g; Fiber: 4g

Pasta e Fagioli

PREP TIME: 10 minutes

COOK TIME: 20 minutes

NUT-FREE, SOY-FREE

SERVES 8

Pasta e fagioli is an Italian dish that literally translates to "pasta and beans." It's a very traditional Italian soup that has origins in peasant homes, where meals were prepared with inexpensive ingredients found on hand or grown on your own land. It's typically made with meat, but we're skipping that part and opting for extra beans to load this soup with protein and fiber.

1 cup ditalini or other small soup pasta

1 tablespoon grapeseed or extra-virgin olive oil

3 carrots, diced

1 medium onion, diced

2 celery stalks, diced

1 teaspoon minced garlic

3 cups low-sodium vegetable broth

1 (16-ounce) jar tomato sauce

1 (15-ounce) can diced tomatoes

1 cup water

1 tablespoon Italian seasoning

½ teaspoon salt

½ teaspoon freshly ground black pepper

1 (15-ounce) can red kidney beans, drained and rinsed

1 (15-ounce) can navy or great northern beans, drained and rinsed

1. Bring a large pot of water to a boil and cook the pasta according to package directions. Drain and set aside.

2. While the pasta is cooking, in a large pot, heat the oil over medium-

high heat. Add the carrots, onion, celery, and garlic and cook for 3 to 4 minutes, until the onions are just translucent.

3. Add the vegetable broth, tomato sauce, tomatoes and their juices, water, Italian seasoning, salt, and pepper. Bring to a boil, then reduce the heat to just below medium and simmer, covered, for 10 to 15 minutes, or until the vegetables are soft.

4. Stir in the beans and pasta and serve.

PER SERVING: Calories: 207; Fat: 3g; Protein: 9g; Carbohydrates: 37g; Fiber: 7g

8

Homemade Staples

Basic Seitan

Meat-Free Pepperoni

Mango Chutney

Cheddar-Style Cheese Sauce

Vegan Mozzarella

Garlic and Herb Tofu Cream Cheese

Everyday Curry Paste

Vegan Mayonnaise

Stir-Fry Sauce

Tofu "Beef" Crumble Three Ways

Basic Seitan

PREP TIME: 15 minutes

COOK TIME: 30 minutes

NUT-FREE, SOY-FREE

SERVES 8

Seitan is a plant-based meat substitute made from wheat gluten and chickpea flour. It can often be found in restaurant and store-bought versions of vegan and vegetarian "meats" or "chicken." Seitan is actually very easy to make, and once you've mastered a basic version, you can customize the seasonings to create any number of flavor creations and uses. Much like tofu, seitan is a blank canvas, so be bold with your seasonings.

1½ cups vital wheat gluten

¼ cup chickpea flour ½

cup nutritional yeast 2

tablespoons paprika 1

teaspoon salt

1 teaspoon curry powder

1 teaspoon ground cumin

1 teaspoon onion powder

1 teaspoon garlic powder

1 teaspoon freshly ground black pepper

1 teaspoon dried oregano

½ teaspoon chili powder

½ teaspoon sumac or ground

cinnamon ½ teaspoon dried thyme

½ teaspoon cornstarch

1½ cups low-sodium vegetable broth 2

tablespoons canola or grapeseed oil

1. In a large bowl, sift together the wheat gluten and chickpea flour. Add the nutritional yeast, paprika, salt, curry powder, cumin, onion powder, garlic powder, black pepper, oregano, chili powder, sumac, thyme, and cornstarch and stir to combine. Make a well in the center of the bowl and pour in the vegetable broth and oil. Mix well to form a dough. Knead the dough in the bowl for 2 to 3 minutes, then set aside to rest for 10 minutes.

2. While the dough is resting, pour 2 inches of water into a large pot with a tight-fitting lid. Place a metal colander in the pot, ensuring the bottom of the colander does not touch the water. Bring the water to a boil, then reduce to a simmer.

3. Knead the dough for 30 seconds, shaping it into a rectangular loaf. Cut into three even pieces and wrap each piece in a sheet of aluminum foil, twisting off the ends to form little packets. Place each packet in the colander over the simmering water and place the lid on top. Steam for 30 minutes.

4. Remove from the pot and let cool for 5 minutes, or until cool enough to handle. Unwrap and cool completely at room temperature. Use as needed or store in an airtight container in the refrigerator for up to 1 week.

INGREDIENT TIP: Vital wheat gluten is the natural protein found in wheat. It gives doughs and breads texture and elasticity and helps bind the other ingredients together. The more activation gluten gets (by kneading or mixing), the stronger and more elastic it becomes, resulting in a better chew. This is important when simulating meats in plant-based cooking because it's the texture and "chew" (or mouthfeel) that makes it satisfying.

PER SERVING: Calories: 173; Fat: 5g; Protein: 23g; Carbohydrates: 12g; Fiber: 4g; Iron 2mg

Meat-Free Pepperoni

PREP TIME: 10 minutes

COOK TIME: 45 minutes

NUT-FREE

SERVES 6

Fennel gives this pepperoni an authentic flavor. It is the perfect complement to Pizza-Night Penne or Pizza Pockets.

1 cup vital wheat gluten

2 teaspoons smoked paprika

2 teaspoons Italian seasoning

1½ teaspoons sugar

1 teaspoon garlic powder

1 teaspoon onion powder

1 teaspoon crushed fennel seeds

1 teaspoon salt

1 teaspoon freshly ground black pepper

½ teaspoon ground mustard

½ to ¾ teaspoon red pepper flakes

½ cup low-sodium vegetable broth

2 tablespoons tomato paste

1 tablespoon canola or grapeseed oil

1 tablespoon tamari or dark soy sauce

1. In a large bowl, combine the wheat gluten, smoked paprika, Italian seasoning, sugar, garlic powder, onion powder, fennel, salt, pepper, ground mustard powder, and red pepper flakes. Make a well in the center of the bowl and add the vegetable broth, tomato paste, oil, and tamari. Combine to form a dough. Knead the dough for 1 to 2 minutes, until rubbery.

2. Halve the dough and roll both pieces into sausage-shaped logs. Wrap each log in aluminum foil, ensuring the foil is overlapped so it doesn't open during cooking, and twist off the ends.

3. In a large pot with a tight-fitting lid, place 2 inches of water. Place a metal colander in the pot, ensuring the bottom of the colander does not touch the water, and bring to a boil. Reduce to a simmer, add the foil-wrapped logs, and cover with the lid. Steam for 45 minutes, checking frequently to ensure the water doesn't evaporate.

4. Let cool at room temperature completely, then refrigerate for at least 1 hour before serving. Store in the refrigerator in an airtight container for up to 6 days.

TECHNIQUE TIP: If you don't have a metal colander, bake these in the oven at 325°F for 90 minutes, turning them over halfway through.

PER SERVING: Calories: 115; Fat: 3g; Protein: 16g; Carbohydrates: 7g; Fiber: 1g; Iron 2mg

Mango Chutney

PREP TIME: 10 minutes

COOK TIME: 15 minutes

GLUTEN-FREE, NUT-FREE, OIL-FREE, ONE POT, SOY-FREE

MAKES ABOUT 2 CUPS

This is a fantastic homemade chutney that takes minutes to make and adds delicious flavor to so many dishes. It's perfect with the Tandoori Jackfruit and Chutney Panini and Curry Penne with Mango Chutney. I even love it as a topping on a black bean burger too. You can swap the fresh mango for 2 cups of frozen mango if needed. Let it thaw at room temperature until soft enough to cut into smaller pieces before cooking.

2 fresh mangos, peeled, pitted, and diced

1 medium onion, diced

½ cup water

1 jalapeño pepper, ribs and seeds removed and finely diced

1 tablespoon brown sugar

1 tablespoon mild yellow curry powder

1 tablespoon freshly squeezed lime juice

½ teaspoon grated ginger

½ teaspoon salt

½ teaspoon freshly ground black pepper

1. In a medium saucepan, combine the mangos, onion, water, jalapeño, brown sugar, curry powder, lime juice, ginger, salt, and pepper and bring to a boil.

2. Reduce the heat to medium-low and simmer, stirring occasionally, until the mixture is thick and most of the liquid has evaporated.

3. Let cool completely, then transfer to an airtight container and store

in the refrigerator for up to 1 month.

TECHNIQUE TIP: You can also preserve this chutney using the traditional canning method in a boiling water bath and it will keep for a year.

VARY IT: No mangos? Swap them for peaches and make a peach chutney instead.

PER SERVING (1 TABLESPOON): Calories: 16; Fat: <1g; Protein: <1g; Carbohydrates: 4g; Fiber: 1g; Iron <1mg

Cheddar-Style Cheese Sauce

PREP TIME: 15 minutes

COOK TIME: 15 minutes

GLUTEN-FREE, NUT-FREE, SOY-FREE

MAKES ABOUT 4 CUPS

I've created and tested close to a dozen different plant-based cheese sauces, and this one is hands-down our family favorite. My kids ask for it on their mac and cheese at least six times a week. What I like most about this recipe is that it uses vegetables to create a creamy, orange-hued sauce instead of processed cheese substitutes. If you follow an oil-free diet, swap the oil in this recipe for aquafaba (the liquid from a can of chickpeas).

2 medium yellow potatoes, peeled and coarsely chopped

2 medium carrots, coarsely chopped

½ cup water

½ cup nutritional yeast

⅓ cup grapeseed or extra-virgin olive oil 1 tablespoon freshly squeezed lemon juice 1 teaspoon salt

¼ teaspoon garlic powder

¼ teaspoon onion powder

1. Bring a large pot of water to a boil and cook the potatoes and carrots until soft, about 10 minutes. Drain and transfer to a high-speed blender or food processor.

2. Add the water, nutritional yeast, oil, lemon juice, salt, garlic powder, and onion powder. Process until smooth and creamy.

3. Store in an airtight container in the refrigerator for up to 5 days.

VARY IT: Elevate your nacho night by turning this cheese sauce into the best vegan queso ever. Add ¼ to ½ teaspoon cayenne pepper and 3 tablespoons pickled jalapeños (with their liquid) to the blender with the other ingredients.

PER SERVING (2 TABLESPOONS): Calories: 36; Fat: 2g; Protein: 1g; Carbohydrates: 3g; Fiber: 1g; Iron <1mg

Vegan Mozzarella

PREP TIME: 10 minutes

COOK TIME: 10 minutes

GLUTEN-FREE, OIL-FREE, SOY-FREE

MAKES ABOUT 1 CUP

Stretchy, melty homemade vegan mozzarella is easier than you think. You can use this cheese in recipes throughout this book, like the Cheesy Summer Squash Flatbreads, Black Bean Meatball Subs, and Pizza-Night Penne.

½ cup raw cashews

1⅓ cups water

¼ cup tapioca starch

Juice of ½ lemon

1 tablespoon apple cider vinegar

1 tablespoon nutritional yeast

½ teaspoon salt

1. Place the cashews in a bowl. Boil about 2 cups water and pour over the cashews. Let stand, covered, for 10 minutes. Drain and discard the water.

2. Add the cashews to a blender with the 1⅓ cups fresh water, tapioca starch, lemon juice, vinegar, nutritional yeast, and salt. Blend until smooth.

3. Pour the cashew mixture into a small saucepan and cook over medium heat, stirring with a spatula or spoon. As it cooks, the mixture will get clumpy. Keep stirring until it becomes a thick, gooey, stretchy ball of cheese. This should take 5 to 6 minutes. Remove from the heat immediately.

4. Use as is for a stretchy, melty cheese, or transfer to an airtight container and refrigerate for at least 1 hour to get a thicker, sliceable

cheese. Store in the refrigerator for up to 6 days or in the freezer for up to 3 months.

INGREDIENT TIP: The trick to this cheese is using tapioca starch (or tapioca flour). Of all the plant-based thickeners, this one gives the most stretch. If you can't find tapioca starch, you can use potato starch or cornstarch, but your cheese won't be as stretchy. It will, however, still solidify into a sliceable cheese.

PER SERVING (2 TABLESPOONS): Calories: 64; Fat: 4g; Protein: 2g; Carbohydrates: 6g; Fiber: 1g; Iron 1mg

Garlic and Herb Tofu Cream Cheese

PREP TIME: 20 minutes

GLUTEN-FREE

MAKES ABOUT 3 CUPS

Cheese was the hardest thing for me to give up, and something tells me I'm not alone here. This has become my go-to vegan cream cheese. It's got a creamy, whipped texture and a rich, tangy garlic flavor, just like the dairy-laden version you'd get at a deli. But best of all, this cream cheese is ready in just under 20 minutes, and there's no lining up on a Sunday morning to get some.

1 (14-ounce) block firm tofu
2 tablespoons chopped fresh flat-leaf parsley or 1 tablespoon dried parsley
2 tablespoons chopped fresh dill or 1 tablespoon dried dill
2 tablespoons freshly squeezed lemon juice
2 tablespoons apple cider vinegar
2 tablespoons melted coconut oil
2 teaspoons minced garlic
1 teaspoon salt
1 teaspoon garlic powder
1 teaspoon onion powder

1. Press the tofu by wrapping it in paper towels and placing it in between two plates weighted down with a heavy object (two cans of beans or tomato sauce work well). Let stand for 10 to 15 minutes.

2. Remove the paper towels, break the tofu into large chunks and add them to a food processor, along with the parsley, dill, lemon juice, vinegar, coconut oil, garlic, salt, garlic powder, and onion powder. Process until smooth.

3. Transfer to an airtight container and refrigerate for up to 1 week.

VARY IT: Swap the parsley and dill for fresh basil and add some nutritional yeast and sun-dried tomatoes (if you use oil-packed ones, you can skip the coconut oil) and turn this into a fabulous sun-dried tomato and basil cream cheese.

PER SERVING (2 TABLESPOONS): Calories: 28; Fat: 2g; Protein: 2g; Carbohydrates: 1g; Fiber: <1g; Iron <1mg

Everyday Curry Paste

PREP TIME: 10 minutes

COOK TIME: 10 minutes

GLUTEN-FREE, NUT-FREE, SOY-FREE

MAKES ABOUT 1 CUP

I love trying store-bought curry pastes. They are easy and convenient and usually not very expensive. There are literally hundreds of different types of curry, ranging from mild to wicked hot, and from smoky to sweet. But it can also be quite fun to make your own. This recipe is a good, everyday mild curry paste that can be used for many dishes in this book.

2 tablespoons grapeseed or extra-virgin olive oil

1 large onion, diced

3 garlic cloves, coarsely chopped

1 red chile pepper, seeded if desired and diced

2-inch piece ginger, peeled and coarsely chopped

2 tablespoons mild curry powder

2 tablespoons tomato paste

1. In a small saucepan, heat the oil on medium-high heat. Add the onion, garlic, red chile, and ginger. Cook for 5 minutes, stirring frequently, until the onion is soft and starting to brown. Add the curry powder and tomato paste and cook for another 3 minutes.

2. Transfer the mixture to a blender or food processor and process until smooth. Cool completely and store in an airtight container in the refrigerator for up to 2 weeks.

PER SERVING (1 TABLESPOON): Calories: 25; Fat: 2g; Protein: <1g; Carbohydrates: 2g; Fiber: 1g; Iron <1mg

Vegan Mayonnaise

PREP TIME: 5 minutes

EASY PREP, GLUTEN-FREE, NO COOK, NUT-FREE

MAKES ABOUT 2 CUPS

Vegan mayonnaise is a game changer for so many dishes. It's an essential condiment, in my opinion, and I'm glad that so many store-bought brands exist for quick and convenient use. I like to balance the convenience of prepackaged with the health benefits of homemade, so I created this vegan mayonnaise that takes just a few minutes to make and has fewer preservatives than store-bought.

½ cup unsweetened soy milk, at room temperature

2 teaspoons apple cider vinegar or freshly squeezed lemon juice

1 teaspoon salt

1 cup canola or grapeseed oil

1. In a blender or food processor, combine the soy milk, vinegar, and salt and blend on low for 5 to 10 seconds. With the blender still running, gradually pour in the oil, increasing the speed once all the oil is added. Continue blending until the mayonnaise has a thick consistency.

2. Adjust the thickness by adding more soy milk to thin it out, or more oil to thicken it, blending after each addition.

3. Store in an airtight container in the refrigerator for up to 4 days.

VARY IT: Switch up your regular mayonnaise by adding a tablespoon or two of sriracha and ½ teaspoon sugar to replicate Japanese-style spicy mayo. Or stir in a spoonful of horseradish and Dijon mustard at the end for a delicious sandwich spread.

PER SERVING (1 TABLESPOON): Calories: 62; Fat: 7g; Protein: <1g; Carbohydrates: <1g; Fiber: 0g; Iron 0mg

Stir-Fry Sauce

PREP TIME: 5 minutes

COOK TIME: 5 minutes

EASY PREP, GLUTEN-FREE, NUT-FREE

MAKES ABOUT ½ CUP

This is a multipurpose stir-fry sauce. It uses a pickled chili sauce called sambal oelek, which is available in the international section of most grocery stores. If you can't find it, just use sriracha or sweet chili sauce instead. You can use this sauce in a variety of dishes throughout this book, including Udon Noodles with Mushrooms and Cabbage, Vegetable Lo Mein, and Broccoli Ramen Stir-Fry.

1 tablespoon cornstarch

4 tablespoons cold water, divided

2 tablespoons tamari

2 tablespoons maple syrup

1 tablespoon apple cider vinegar

1 tablespoon freshly squeezed lime juice

1 tablespoon tahini

2 teaspoons sesame oil

1 teaspoon brown sugar

1½ teaspoons grated ginger

2 garlic cloves, minced

½ teaspoon sambal oelek or other hot sauce

1. In a medium bowl, dissolve the cornstarch in 2 tablespoons of cold water. Add the tamari, remaining 2 tablespoons of water, maple syrup, vinegar, lime juice, tahini, sesame oil, brown sugar, ginger, garlic, and sambal oelek and whisk to combine.

2. Transfer the sauce to a small saucepan and simmer over medium heat for about 5 minutes, stirring continuously, until the sauce

thickens. Remove from the heat.

3. Use right away, or transfer to an airtight container and refrigerate for up to 1 week.

PER SERVING (1 TABLESPOON): Calories: 45; Fat: 2g; Protein: 1g; Carbohydrates: 6g; Fiber: <1g; Iron <1mg

Tofu "Beef" Crumble Three Ways

PREP TIME: 5 minutes

COOK TIME: 30 minutes

GLUTEN-FREE, NUT-FREE

MAKES ABOUT 3 CUPS

Crumbled tofu is a versatile substitute for ground meat, and it's much healthier than store-bought versions. I've included three of my most-used versions—Tex-Mex-style, Korean barbecue-style, and Bolognese-style, all of which will come in very handy for recipes in this book.

For Tex-Mex-style tofu

1 tablespoon canola or grapeseed oil

1 teaspoon tamari

1 tablespoon chili powder

1 teaspoon ground cumin

1 teaspoon garlic powder

1 teaspoon paprika

½ teaspoon dried oregano

½ teaspoon onion

powder ¼ teaspoon salt

¼ teaspoon freshly ground black pepper

1 (14-ounce) block extra-firm tofu, drained and pressed

For Korean barbecue–style tofu

1 tablespoon sesame oil

¼ cup tamari

2 teaspoons minced garlic

¼ cup packed brown sugar

¼ teaspoon ground ginger

¼ teaspoon red pepper flakes

1 (14-ounce) block extra-firm tofu, drained and pressed

For Bolognese-style tofu

1 tablespoon canola or grapeseed oil

1 teaspoon tamari

1 tablespoon dried oregano

1 tablespoon dried basil

¼ teaspoon red pepper flakes (or more if you want it

spicy) ½ teaspoon smoked paprika

½ teaspoon garlic powder

½ teaspoon onion powder

¼ teaspoon salt

¼ teaspoon ground pepper

1 (14-ounce) block extra-firm tofu, drained and pressed

1. Preheat the oven to 350°F. Line a rimmed baking sheet with parchment paper.

2. In a small bowl, combine the ingredients (except the tofu) for your chosen seasoning style. Mix until they form a paste. Set aside.

3. In a large bowl, crumble the tofu into small chunks. Toss with the spice paste until all the tofu pieces are coated. Spread the tofu onto the prepared baking sheet in an even layer.

4. Bake for 30 minutes, tossing the crumble every 10 minutes.

5. Use right away, or cool completely and store in an airtight container in the refrigerator for up to 5 days or in the freezer for up to 3 months.

Tex-Mex-style

PER SERVING (½ CUP): Calories: 100; Fat: 6g; Protein: 8g; Carbohydrates: 4g; Fiber: 2g; Iron 2mg

Korean barbecue–style

PER SERVING (½ CUP): Calories: 134; Fat: 6g; Protein: 8g; Carbohydrates: 12g; Fiber: 1g; Iron 2mg

Bolognese-style

PER SERVING (½ CUP): Calories: 96; Fat: 6g; Protein: 7g; Carbohydrates: 3g; Fiber: 1g; Iron 2mg

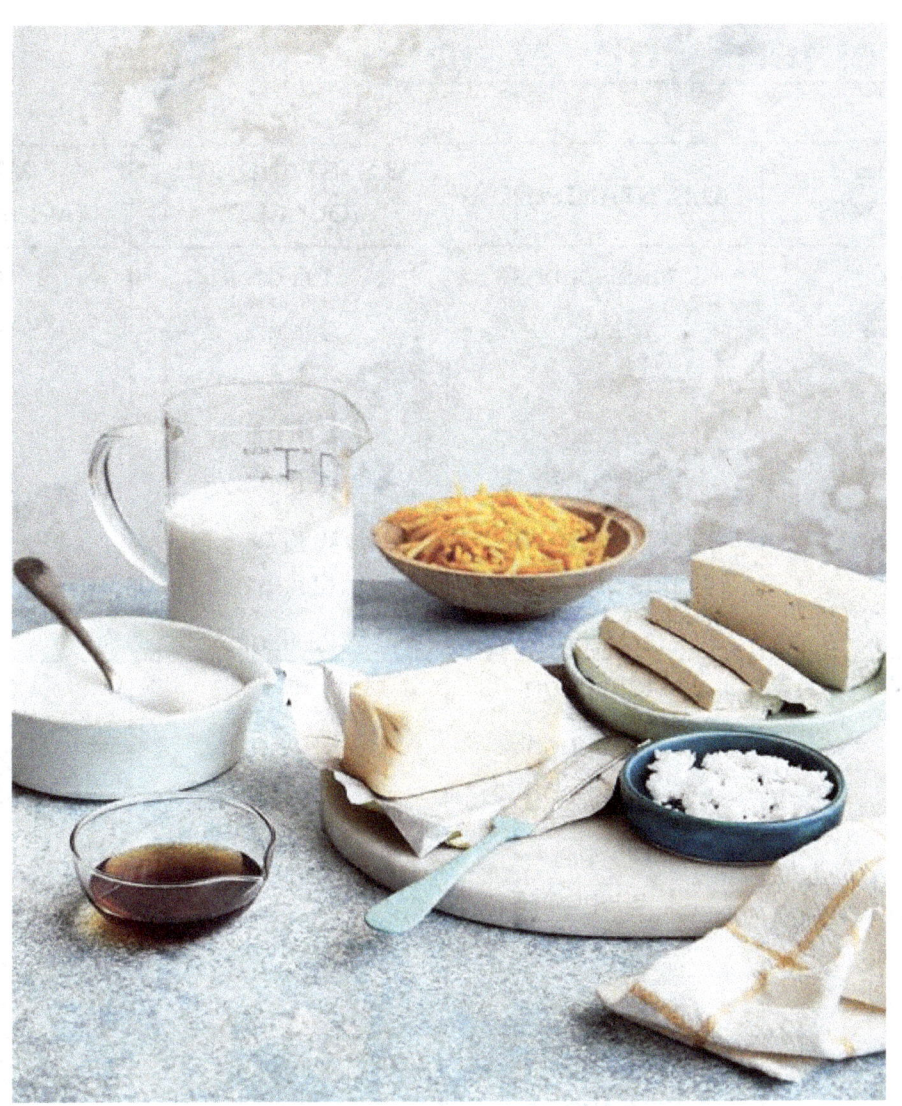

Measurement Conversions

VOLUME EQUIVALENTS	U.S. STANDARD	U.S. STANDARD (OUNCES)	METRIC (APPROXIMATE)
LIQUID	2 tablespoons	1 fl. oz.	30 mL
	¼ cup	2 fl. oz.	60 mL
	½ cup	4 fl. oz.	120 mL
	1 cup	8 fl. oz.	240 mL
	1½ cups	12 fl. oz.	355 mL
	2 cups or 1 pint	16 fl. oz.	475 mL
	4 cups or 1 quart	32 fl. oz.	1 L
	1 gallon	128 fl. oz.	4 L
DRY	⅛ teaspoon	—	0.5 mL
	¼ teaspoon	—	1 mL
	½ teaspoon	—	2 mL
	¾ teaspoon	—	4 mL
	1 teaspoon	—	5 mL
	1 tablespoon	—	15 mL
	¼ cup	—	59 mL
	⅓ cup	—	79 mL
	½ cup	—	118 mL
	⅔ cup	—	156 mL
	¾ cup	—	177 mL
	1 cup	—	235 mL
	2 cups or 1 pint	—	475 mL
	3 cups	—	700 mL
	4 cups or 1 quart	—	1 L
	½ gallon	—	2 L
	1 gallon	—	4 L

OVEN TEMPERATURES

FAHRENHEIT	CELSIUS (APPROXIMATE)
250°F	120°C
300°F	150°C
325°F	165°C
350°F	180°C
375°F	190°C
400°F	200°C
425°F	220°C
450°F	230°C

WEIGHT EQUIVALENTS

U.S. STANDARD	METRIC (APPROXIMATE)
½ ounce	15 g
1 ounce	30 g
2 ounces	60 g
4 ounces	115 g
8 ounces	225 g
12 ounces	340 g
16 ounces or 1 pound	455 g

CPSIA information can be obtained
at www.ICGtesting.com
Printed in the USA
BVHW011338210621
610122BV00003B/181